I USED TO HAVE CANCER

HOW I FOUND MY OWN WAY BACK TO HEALTH

JAMES TEMPLETON

SQUAREONE
PUBLISHERS
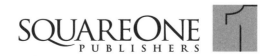

COVER DESIGNER: Jeannie Rosado
IN-HOUSE EDITOR: Marie Caratozzolo
TYPESETTER: Gary A. Rosenberg

Square One Publishers
115 Herricks Road
Garden City Park, NY 11040
(516) 535-2010 • (877) 900-BOOK
www.squareonepublishers.com

The information and advice contained in this book are based upon the research and the personal and professional experiences of the authors. They are not intended as a substitute for consulting with a health care professional. The publisher and author are not responsible for any adverse effects or consequences resulting from the use of any of the suggestions, preparations, or procedures discussed in this book. All matters pertaining to your physical health should be supervised by a health care professional. It is a sign of wisdom, not cowardice, to seek a second or third opinion.

Library of Congress Cataloging-in-Publication Data
Names: Templeton, James William, author.
Title: I used to have cancer : how I found my own way back to health / James
  Templeton.
Description: Garden City Park, NY : Square One Publishers, 2019. | Includes
  bibliographical references and index.
Identifiers: LCCN 2019007661 | ISBN 9780757004780
Subjects: LCSH: Templeton, James William,—Health. |
  Melanoma—Patients—Biography. | Cancer—Patients—Biography. |
  Cancer—Patients—Nutrition. | Cancer—Patients—Psychology.
Classification: LCC RC280.M37 T46 2019 | DDC 616.99/4770092 [B] —dc23
LC record available at https://lccn.loc.gov/2019007661

Printed in the United States of America

10   9   8   7   6   5   4   3   2   1

Contents

*This book is lovingly dedicated
to the beautiful Ann Louise Gittleman,
with whom I've been fortunate enough
to spend the best years of my life.*

Acknowledgments

I felt alone as I lay helplessly in the hospital, but it turned out that it wasn't so. I am eternally grateful to the teachers and way-showers who rescued me and helped me along my crazy journey back to health. My sincere thanks go out to every one of you.

To the late Ron Sumter, a preacher from my hometown of Huntsville, Texas, who spurred me with his unorthodox prayer to "fight like hell." It was exactly the fresh spark I needed as I lay dying. And to Dirk Benedict whose book *Confessions of a Kamikaze Cowboy* was an answer to my desperate prayer. His story and words awakened in me a newfound hope, which saved my life, opened my eyes to new possibilities of healing, and thrust me onto the most amazing rollercoaster ride. Were it not for the book review written by Len Kasten, which was delivered to me at my hospital door by an old college friend, Ron Davidge, I would not have known about Dirk's book and, likely, would not be alive to tell my story.

To Michio and Aveline Kushi of the Kushi Institute, for their extraordinary knowledge, teaching, and guidance. To Ed Esko and Charles Millman, for their many kindness, support, and valuable advice. To Alex and Gale Jack, for their friendship, support, and countless fine meals. To all the men and women with whom I spent time at the Kushi Institute, who meant more to me than they will ever know. The times I spent there were enormously healing in more ways than one, and I will treasure those days forever.

To Dr. Linus Pauling and Dr. Matthias Rath, whose extraordinary work and research lit the way for me and opened up avenues of healing I never dreamed existed. To the late Dr. Anthony Sattilaro, may he rest in peace, for the words of inspiration and courage found in his work. To Dr. Hazel Parcells—teacher of teachers—for all her advice, which I still revere. This red-haired Irish woman who lived to the age of 106 was one of a kind. She earned her knowledge the hard way. To Dr. Hermann Bueno, renowned parasitologist, who demonstrated to me the invisible world of parasites and solved one of the greatest mysteries of my condition. To Ron Koetzsch for his invaluable guidance. To my ardent supporters Dr. Lee Cowden and Doug Kaufmann, who have been fighting the good fight for many years. To Dr. Roy Speiser, the water doctor, and Dr. Diane Romeo, for their friendship and breakthroughs on clean water. And to my personal health heroes: mercury-free dental pioneer Dr. Hal Huggins, microscopy expert Dr. Bob Bradford, and Eddie Aldworth (a gentleman's gentleman), who took me under his wing.

Without the support of family and friends, I would not be where I am today. To my ancestors from whom I inherited the fighting spirit they exemplified—I've called upon that courage when I've been against the ropes and I've tried to make you proud. To the greatest sister in the world, Judy Heath; her terrific husband, Levi Heath; and my beloved nephews, James and Shanon Heath—I can't thank you enough for all the good times we've shared over the years! It has meant the world to me. To my precious daughter, Carol, my reason for living; and her husband, Blaise, who has made her life complete. To Carol's mother, for raising our daughter through the rough times. And to my grandson, Caleb, who continues to fill my heart with joy and wonder. I look forward to many more discoveries with you at my side.

To my close friends Herb Shapiro and Paula Breen, without whose support and friendship through the years—and at the most precarious points in my life—I would be lost. To Allen Goehrs, for the inspiration and opportunity he and his father gave me at a critical point in my life's journey; Bill Carmichael, my compadre and running buddy, who saw me through some of the toughest times; and Randy Pachar, for believing in me enough to give me a chance.

To Ann Louise Gittleman, tireless health warrior, who continues to lead the way in discovering new avenues of health and wellness. Thank you for being by my side. You are one of a kind, and I cherish your love and concern.

I couldn't have taken the time to write a book if my primary businesses weren't in the best of hands. My deepest gratitude goes to Stuart Gittleman, for his extraordinary project management skills and his unwavering support. And to my very capable behind-the-scenes crew that spans all time zones of the continental US, and of which I am most proud: Carol Templeton (my daughter and savvy Marketing Manager), Matt Carnegie, Lonnie Wollin (awesome accountant/attorney), Jan Cramer, Olga

Schwedland, Dave Stetzelberger, Rhonda Willette-Watts, Bonnie Cerrillo, Kea Fisher, Liz Patton, Tracy St. Peter, Bianca Hernandez, Kathleen Sullivan, and Emily Carmichael. To Maria Lowe, one of our most cherished personal chefs from years gone by, and her amazing macro meals. You rock! And to Teresa Pfaff, our current personal chef, who now keeps me happily fed and nourished!

This book would not have come about if not for the expert guidance of Rudy Shur, CEO of Square One Publishers. Rudy's personal dedication to spreading the word about all forms of healing is unique among publishers. Rudy, thank you for believing in me. And kudos to the very capable Anthony Pomes and his marketing expertise! Thank you also to Rhonda Burns, a kindred spirit and able cowriter who helped me turn my life story into written words.

I carry with me the inspiring words of John Denver and the music that helped to heal my heart. The memories of my heroes along the way—John Wayne, Don Meredith, Jack LaLanne—men who were extraordinary in their own lives and careers, remain a part of me. They don't make 'em like they used to!

I wrote this book for the countless men, women, and children with a life-changing diagnosis who are searching for hope and healing. May you each find your door to hope and run, not walk, through it! And to the amazing doctors and bold health practitioners who are setting aside their fears and fighting to find and deliver a natural approach to healing for all, I send my heart-felt wish: Godspeed!

One final note: A number of names have been changed to protect the privacy of these individuals.

Foreword

J ames Templeton is indeed a "born storyteller." And his story is an important one.

There is a saying within conventional medicine that "the plural of anecdote (a fancy word for "story") is not evidence." Nevertheless, such stories are important. They make us realize that unusual things are possible. And if more people engage in such "possibility" thinking, then more things may become possible.

I have worked with people with cancer challenges in many different ways since 1973, first as a medical student exploring nutritional therapies, then as a young holistic medical doctor exploring alternative cancer therapies, and ultimately as a medical oncologist (having done six years of hospital-based residency and fellowship training after twelve years in practice of holistic/integrative medicine). Early in this process, I had the insight that viewing cancer as a teacher who tells us about how we've been living our lives can be far more productive than battling it as an enemy.

In this book, Mr. Templeton, after telling the engaging story of his very enlightening journey with melanoma, reached the conclusion that having cancer helped teach him how to live fully and healthfully. He has since devoted his life to helping others deal with similar challenges, providing information, products, and inspiration so that others may find what he found.

The first step in dealing with an "incurable" cancer is believing that vibrant cancer-free health can be obtained. If one doesn't believe this, then the cancer truly is "incurable." My advice to people facing significant cancer challenges has long been to find therapies and practitioners that inspire confidence. Confidence is fundamental to healing from cancer. Fear is deadly. It activates the sympathetic (fight/flight/freeze) nervous system, which deactivates the parasympathetic nervous system, which

controls the digestive and immune functions, both of which are fundamental to healing from cancer.

Another important lesson that comes through in this book is the
importance of trusting one's intuition. Every person's path to healing will
be a little different from everyone else's. Certainly there are over-arching
principles that apply to all, but the details can be quite different. We don't
yet have the science to reliably guide us to cures of advanced stages of
many types of cancer, and intuition may well be our best guide. It certainly served James Templeton well. He knew instinctively, for instance,
that macrobiotics was to play a major role in his recovery, even before he
had learned anything about it.

Through his story, discover Templeton's principles of healthy living.
He can inspire a confidence in the people he counsels that no oncologist or
scientist can. James Templeton has succeeded in staying well despite the
odds, which were strongly stacked against him. You can, too.

Dwight L. McKee, MD, CNS, ABIHM
Board certified in Medical Oncology,
Nutrition, Integrative and Holistic Medicine

1

Living the American Dream

*"We are stronger in the places
we have been broken."*

—ERNEST HEMINGWAY

It's funny how life can throw major curve balls at you when you least expect it. When I was in my early thirties, I absolutely believed that I was at the top of my game. I was living the American dream—had a family of my own, a nice house on a small farm, and a number of successful businesses in my East Texas hometown. Everything was going great. I guess you might say I had life by the tail. Little did I know that although I had overcome a number of challenges in my life at that point, my biggest challenge was yet to come.

The day started out like most others, but I had no idea a new curve ball was headed my way. I got up before dawn to go on my morning run. It wasn't so much that I liked waking up early to pound the pavement, but I was addicted to it. Running was my way of keeping a tight rein on what I considered to be a family curse. My mother died before I was two, so I really don't remember her. I never had a chance to get to know my grandfather, either. He died at the ripe young age of thirty-six, many years before I was even born. I was told he died because of a bad heart. My younger stepbrother died at the age of eight, never really getting to enjoy life. But when my father—Daddy—died unexpectedly of a heart attack when he was only forty-six, it affected me deeply, unlike anything that had ever affected me before. I became enraged that life had dealt me yet another blow.

I'm deeply grateful for my sister, Judy, who is two and a half years older than I am. Throughout the difficult years of growing up, she was my guardian angel. I don't know what I would have done without her. To this day, there has never been an unkind word between us. Judy has been the thread that has held our family together over the years and provided me with the stability I needed.

While I knew that it wasn't possible to prevent every premature death, I sure as hell didn't want to go to an early grave the way my father and grandfather did—so I did the one thing that I thought could help. I ran. I ran every chance I got—in the pouring rain, in the sweltering heat, and in the bitter cold. Whether I was home or on the road, I ran. I realize now I was running from fear. But back then, running was my way of proving to myself that I had found a way to sidestep my family's curse—heart disease. Running was also my time for meditation, the time when I did my deepest thinking. I felt virtuous, proud, wise . . . and sometimes even invincible when I was running.

"It's great to be alive!" I thought as I darted out the front door and down the dusty farm road. Even though the sun was not yet up, I could tell it was going to be one of those summer days when rivers of sweat would soon be running down my face and trickling down my neck and back. I could already feel my shirt starting to cling to my back.

Jumping the railroad tracks, I continued running until I reached the smooth pavement of the rural highway. I ran along the road with the woods on either side. On a warm night in East Texas, the woods sounded rowdier than a busy bar—with crickets singing, owls hooting, and frogs bellowing on the banks of a nearby pond. But when the locusts and song-birds take over just before daylight, you couldn't find a better symphony anywhere. It was my favorite time of day . . . once I was up and around, that is. About the only vehicle I'd ever encounter during those early morn-ing runs was an occasional log truck. As the long, empty vehicle rumbled by on its way to pick up the daily harvest of tall pines or post oaks, I'd enjoy the brief rush of air left in its wake.

The path I followed on my morning runs led me past the visual reminders of the losses in my life. Less than four miles from my front door as the crow flies was Black Jack Cemetery. This prominent local landmark is where many of my family members were buried. It had become my touchstone. Circling the little church there, I glanced over at my daddy's grave. I always felt closer to him when I ran, believing he would have been gratified to know what I had accomplished. Fifteen miles or so from my house was yet another cemetery where many other family members had been laid to rest. I was proud and felt privileged to live where generations of my ancestors had settled. They were part of the bricks and mortar that built the great State of Texas.

I come from a long line of fighters. Some fought not only in the War of 1812, but also in the war for Texas independence some twenty-four years later. My ancestors had come to Texas in 1832 when Mexico was giving land grants to foreigners. It wasn't long before the Texans outnumbered the Mexicans. Then the inevitable happened—the Mexican government's attempt to regulate the growing Texas communities led to outright rebellion. So when General Sam Houston called for a volunteer militia to fight for Texas' independence after the battle at the Alamo, my ancestors were right there with him in the cause.

One April afternoon in 1836, General Houston and his group of about eight hundred Texans launched a surprise attack at the Battle of San Jacinto near present-day Houston. It was there that they thoroughly routed the Mexican army of nearly twice as many men, led by General Santa Anna. Seems they figured out that attacking the enemy during their daily siesta would give them a real surprise advantage. I've always admired my family's fighting spirit, ingenuity, and just plain good horse sense, often against incredible odds. As it turned out, I would need to tap into these same qualities very shortly . . . in the fight for my own life.

My sister Judy and I agree that we couldn't have asked for a better father. His early death came as a real shock to all of us who knew and loved him. Though we felt cheated by his death, we recognized that the time we had with him was precious. Daddy never had an unkind word for anyone. He wasn't what folks considered wealthy, but he was a talented man who was rich in all the things that matter—kindness, character, and loyalty. He was also rich in the love of his family. A machinist by trade, my father could build or fix anything. He took meticulous care in all that he did and of everything he owned, from the roof on our house to our lawn, which he kept perfectly manicured. By his example, he taught me to do the same. Keeping my house, my car, and all my belongings in tip-top shape is something that has always been important to me.

Daddy would take me to my little league and football games, and he even helped coach as often as he could. We'd watch baseball games on TV in the summer and the Houston Oilers and Dallas Cowboys during football season. He'd also take me hunting every once in a while, as was more or less expected of the men of that time and place. I looked forward to spending those times with him. We'd mostly just sit quietly in the deer stand on those early mornings in the woods. Though we'd be on the lookout for a big buck, more often than naught, it was a doe and one or two of her little ones that would walk by. We'd sit in silence and let them pass, and they never knew we were there.

Most folks said my daddy never really got over my mother's death and I thought that was probably true. Lynna Faye, his first wife and my mother, was known as one of the prettiest girls in town. I'm told she was happy-go-lucky, musically inclined, and even played the violin in her college orchestra. I've often wondered how my life would have been different had she lived and if she would have taught me how to play an instrument, too.

When I was four years old, my father remarried. My stepmother, Dorothy, helped raise my sister and me, along with our younger stepbrother, Melvin. "Mama" as we called her, and the only mother I ever really knew, saw to it that I had plenty of responsibility in our busy household. She even taught me how to iron, and, to this day, I still iron my own clothes. Mama was disciplined and strict, but kindhearted. She was always there for us if we needed her. I had no idea how important that would be to me in the years to come.

When Mama was pregnant with Melvin, she was injured in a car accident and underwent x-rays as a result. When Melvin was born with mental and physical disabilities, we often wondered if the accident or the x-rays may have been the cause. As a family, we all shared the responsibility of taking care of Melvin, who required round-the-clock attention. He died when he was only eight years old. It was a very sad time for all of us, and especially hard on Mama and Daddy. We felt like he never had a chance to enjoy life.

I was seventeen years old and a senior in high school when my father died. That Sunday afternoon, I was working as a carpet layer's helper. I remember being touched that he had made a sack lunch for me to take when I left the house that morning. That afternoon, he had gone to a union meeting. After the meeting, as he was walking down the stairs to leave, he suffered a heart attack.

When I got the news that my dad had been taken to the hospital, I dropped everything and rushed there. Running in the main door of the emergency room, I asked the woman at the desk where I could find my father. She asked his name, looked through her records, and then said, "He's gone."

"He's gone home?" I asked, hope rising.

"No, he's dead," she said. Just like that. No fanfare. No "I'm sorry to tell you this, but . . ." No "Sit down while I get the doctor on duty." Just, "He's dead." The words struck me like a hammer and I crumpled to the floor.

There had been no chance to say good-bye to him. Without any warning at all, he was gone. There was nothing to be done. There was no place to go except home. I felt a rush of hurt and pain that swept over me. And I was angry—so angry that when I got home, I put my fist through the hallway wall. Never before had I felt such intense emotion. He was too young to die! It wasn't fair to him . . . or to those of us he left behind.

We all deal differently with pain, of course. Like it or not, death forces us to go through the pain of the grieving process. Some people have the benefit of a "pre-grieving" stage, which often occurs when a loved one suffers a long, painful illness and death comes as a welcome release. But with the sudden, unexpected death of my father, I was thrown head-on into the "shock" stage of grieving, see-sawing between disbelief and unbearable emotional pain. I couldn't imagine life without Daddy. I didn't want to. I had lost too many of my family too soon, and I was sick of it. My father's death was the straw that broke the camel's back for me.

No one gives us a script to follow during these life-changing events. So in my attempt to numb the pain that didn't seem to stop, I did what a lot of people do. I coped with my grief through escape, which included self-medication—plenty of partying, overindulging in food, and, I'll admit, too many beers on too many occasions. The momentary escape from the pain was a welcome relief. And with my daddy not around to keep me in line, I partied my way through the final days of high school. I did, however, manage to continue working on weekends. I had to in order to have the spending money I wanted and needed.

I went to college because my stepmother said it was what my father would have wanted me to do. Sitting in class, though, I confess that I really didn't see the point. The truth was that I thought life was too short to take things so seriously. It seemed to me that a lot of the people I met in college were far too serious, especially many of the professors. In my opinion, partying was where it was at. I hid my pain by trying to be the life of the party.

I started out taking business courses, but soon found them boring. So I began taking criminal justice courses instead. Perhaps watching too many cop movies gave me the idea that being a detective and solving murder mysteries would somehow be exciting. But all it took was one class visit to a state prison to figure out that I wanted nothing more to do with this criminal justice thing.

Finally, I had enough. What a bunch of hogwash it all was, I thought. At that point in my life, I figured I would be lucky if I lived to be thirty, so why was I bothering with college? What was the point? No doubt about it, I had a real what's-the-use attitude. The truth was that I'd had enough of all the pain and the stress of the losses in my short life, and I just wanted it all to go away.

I may not have been a detective, but I did figure out that college wasn't for me. I dropped out after my third year, without even knowing what direction to take next. Not having any guidance from my dad, I knew I'd have to figure it out on my own. I definitely knew how to party hard and, fortunately, I had no problem working just as hard at whatever job I had. When my father was alive, he had worked plenty hard to provide the things our family needed. So I knew from a young age that I would have to work to make money for anything that I might need or want. And besides, I liked the idea of having nice things. A shiny new Chevy pick-up truck didn't sound so bad to me either.

I had been working part-time all through college at a gas station owned by a young entrepreneur named Randy Pachar. Many weekends, I also worked digging ditches for a landscape irrigation company owned by Allen Goehrs and his father. But after I dropped out of college, I traded sitting in a classroom for working full-time for Allen and his dad. I learned real quick that I didn't want to dig ditches the rest of my life, especially in the hot Texas sun. But I did learn to appreciate Allen and his dad's business sense, the things they had, and the level of success they had reached. I wanted the same things. I knew I needed to figure out a career path for myself. Allen became my mentor and I eagerly learned everything he could teach me about his business—a self-directed trade school, you might say. By watching him, my ambition, which I didn't even realize I had until then, kicked in. I began thinking about how someday I might own my own business, too.

I dated here and there, but nothing very serious until I met Mellisa. Pretty and smart, Mellisa had majored in both English and Home Economics, graduating at the top of her class. One invitation to a meal of her home-cooked lasagna was proof positive that there's something to that old saying about the way to a man's heart being through his stomach. By this time, I was twenty-four. Most of my friends were settling down and I figured it was time for me to settle down, too. Six months or so after I popped the question, Mellisa and I had a big church wedding and a beautiful reception at her parents' house. I was happy to be with her—and a little happiness was just what I was looking for.

After we were married, we rented a one-bedroom apartment in Houston. I was working for Allen, and Mellisa, although she had a teaching degree, worked for an engineering and construction company that specialized in designing and building oil refineries. Mellisa stayed fit and trim by running, and we'd often run together. The years of partying and not caring what I ate had caused me to put on a few extra pounds, and I knew that the exercise would be good for me.

Randy, my boss at the gas station I worked at in college, was only three or four years older than I was, but had already found success as a young entrepreneur. One day while I was at work, I mentioned to Randy that I'd love to own a gas station like he did, and if he ever wanted to sell the station to let me know. I'm glad I did because after he put the station up for sale, he asked if I was still interested in buying it. I sure was! I talked it over with Mellisa and we decided to go for it. So we bought the exact gas station where I had worked. The dream to own my own business was kindled, and I quickly set about making my dream come to life.

Based on my taking over the station, it wasn't long before Mellisa was able to quit her job. We worked together to build up our business. She handled the bookkeeping and filled in behind the counter and anywhere else she was needed. I handled the inventory, hiring, and pretty much everything else. But that was only the beginning. Just like Randy had done, we took the money we made from our gas station and bought another one, and eventually I built (from scratch) the *Supr Sak* gas and convenience store in Huntsville, just north of Houston. One thing led to another and before we knew it, we had three. Once we had mastered and maintained a number of successful *Supr Sak* locations, we felt there would be no stopping us. At least, that was the plan.

As part of our new-found ambition, Mellisa used her superb cooking skills to build up a successful catering business. I joined a couple of other friends in the oil field equipment rental business. They handled the sales for a special type of pump for oil rigs, while I maintained and delivered the equipment to different regions of Texas during the oil boom.

Sometimes a pump was needed in an emergency situation, so I'd drive all night to deliver it. Seemed like all I did was work.

Mellisa and I settled into a routine. We built a house on the farm southeast of Huntsville that I had inherited—a gentleman's ranch, you might say. We had a few cattle, some hogs, and dogs and cats. We were very busy. It seemed like we worked from daylight to dark and then some. We had been married over five years before our daughter, Carol, came along. I had no idea that a blonde-haired baby girl with beautiful, bouncy curls could turn my heart inside out the way she did, but there was no denying that she had me wrapped around her little finger from the get-go. She was the best part of my day. I was on cloud nine and living the American Dream. What else could I ask for?

But there was always that nagging worry in the back of my mind. The older I got, the more I began to wonder if I might be destined to die of a heart attack like my grandfather and my daddy. The last thing I wanted to do was to die early and leave my wife behind and my daughter fatherless as I had been. So in addition to my regular daily runs, I began working out even more at the local gym in an effort to make myself as fit as possible.

I remember learning about the famous runner, Jim Fixx. His fanaticism about running was spurred by his own father's death at age thirty-five. Concern about his hereditary predisposition to heart disease led him to give up his habit of smoking two packs of cigarettes a day, shed his excess pounds, and eventually become this country's "guru" of running. His best-selling book, *The Complete Book of Running*, made him a millionaire. He was credited with starting America's fitness revolution as he preached the gospel that active people live longer. His story resonated with me. He was the expert! And I followed his example.

I went from occasionally running with my wife to running every chance I got. It became an obsession. I discovered what the runner's high was all about. I would challenge myself to run up a hill just to feel the exhilaration at the top and the ease of running downhill. I'd try to run in the cool of the morning, knowing that if I didn't, I'd be sweating it out in the hot afternoon. I learned how to push myself when I wanted to quit. I might run only five to eight miles on weekdays, but on weekends, I'd enjoy a satisfying run, often up to eighteen miles. I wasn't the fastest guy in town, but I held my own in local races and half-marathons.

I joined up with my good friend Bill Carmichael, who was as much into running as I was, and we'd run as often as we could. My whole life soon became focused around working and running. I was caught up in my own desire to make a good living and to maintain my health based on what the experts told me. With every step I ran, I believed I was staving off my own premature death just like Jim Fixx, the Running Guru, recommended. I was determined to do all I could to stay fit and healthy and out of an early grave. Running kept me disciplined and taught me an important life's lesson—that every little challenge is broken down into one step at a time. That's as easy and as hard as every task is.

Back on my early morning run that day, I found myself nearly lost in thought as I glanced at my watch. No time to spare. As I headed back to the house, I mentally checked off the tasks I needed to handle first thing that morning. Check to see if we had enough petrol at the station to get through the weekend . . . check our grocery inventory numbers . . . the usual. Keeping everything running smoothly was a full-time job. And living on the farm and tending to it assured there was barely time for anything else. After a full day's work in town, there were cows and hogs to feed and dog runs to clean when I got home. And it seemed like there was always a fence to mend somewhere.

No light on in the kitchen meant Mellisa was still asleep. Baby Carol must still be asleep, too, I chuckled, or the whole house would be awake. I was thirty-two years old. I had my own home, successful businesses, and a beautiful family. And I believed that by running and keeping myself fit and following the advice of the Running Guru, I had figured out how to sidestep my genetic predisposition to an early death. "Life is good," I thought again. "I've got it made."

It was 5:30 AM by the time I finished my run. After a quick shower, I jumped in my truck and headed to town to open up one of our stores. I'd grab breakfast later in the morning at the restaurant down the street. There was a time when I'd typically load up on bacon, eggs, and anything else I wanted, thinking that the calories I burned when running would cancel out the calories I consumed. But after I discovered a book called *Eat to Win: The Sports Nutrition Bible* by Robert Haas, I changed my diet to include more vegetables and very little protein. I'd fill up at salad bars at local restaurants, work out three days a week at the gym, and run every chance I got.

Over time, I began to notice that I was feeling more tired than usual and had more than my fair share of colds, flus, and sinus problems. My solution was simple—I had to push myself even harder. And that's exactly what I did.

The familiar drive to town that day left my mind free to wander. Mellisa would be coming to the office to handle the bookkeeping later that morning, so we'd have a little time together. It wasn't exactly the quality time we had when we were first married, but it was the best we could do. I guess we were like a lot of married couples. Both of us had our hands full as we maintained the businesses, the farm, and our family life. There wasn't much time left over for anything else. Working together as a married couple can be a challenge and put stress on the relationship from time to time. We were working seven days a week, with seldom a day off.

I pulled into the parking lot of the *Supr Sak*. As I let myself in the store, I turned on the lights just as the street lights faded. The sun was up and it was going to be another scorcher. A couple of hours later, with our employees busy at work and the store humming along, I stopped to pour myself a cup of coffee and prop my feet up on my desk in the back office. Opening the newspaper, the headline hit me like a ton of bricks.

"JAMES F. FIXX DIES JOGGING;
AUTHOR ON RUNNING WAS 52."

I was in a state of pure shock! Jim Fixx had died of a heart attack . . . while he was jogging! At that moment, little did I know that his death would ultimately save my own life.

2

The Words No One
Wants to Hear

*"Hope doesn't require a massive chain where heavy links
of logic hold it together. A thin wire will do . . . just strong
enough to get us through the night until the winds die down."*
—Charles R. Swindoll

The bottom dropped from my stomach the way it did when I was a kid on a roller coaster holding on for dear life. Jim Fixx, the famous runner and fitness guru, dead at age fifty-two? Heart attack while jogging? Was this some kind of a joke? A bad dream?

Obviously, learning of someone dying from a heart attack wasn't new to me. I had experienced it in my own family and even had a friend who, at the age of thirty-one, got out of his pickup truck, fell over, and died right there in the parking lot. But I knew better, didn't I? After all, Jim Fixx, the Running Guru, had shown me how to avoid the very type of death that I most dreaded. I was dedicated to running, staying fit, and doing all the right things. My dedication to health even made me feel virtuous. I felt protected from the fate that I had feared. But there it was, undeniable, in black and white. The headline read, "JIM FIXX DEAD." I sure didn't expect this.

The coffee got cold in my cup as I sat there trying to process what I'd just read. I had followed Jim's advice, believing he had the answer to preventing an early death from heart disease. I had devoted all my energy and spare time to running. And for what? That old familiar feeling came rushing back. If Jim Fixx could die of a heart attack, could it happen to me, too? Had I wasted my time on the wrong solution?

I was thirty-two years old, only four years younger than my grandfather was when he died. Maybe I was kidding myself that I was as fit and healthy as I thought I was. Maybe Jim Fixx didn't have the answer after all. I sure didn't like going to the doctor any more than the next guy, but I figured I'd better go for a checkup just to be sure my heart was in good shape. What I needed was one of those stress tests, I thought to myself. Yeah, that's what I would do. I had too much at stake, with a wife and a daughter I didn't want to leave behind . . . along with all my hopes and dreams.

The busy-ness of life had gotten in the way, but after a couple months, I managed to schedule a cardiac stress test with a local internist who had been referred to me by my family doctor. When I got to the office, and after sitting in the waiting room for what seemed like forever, a nurse brought me into the exam room and instructed me to take off my shirt. Then the doctor came in and hooked me up to a hefty number of monitors and wires.

"The electrocardiographic test," he explained, "is designed to test heart function before, during, and after a controlled period of increasingly strenuous exercise." At his instruction, I stepped on a treadmill and submitted to his battery of tests. He gradually increased the speed of the treadmill until I was running. He measured my heart rate and recovery time at varying intervals. When he was finished, he told me to get dressed and meet him in his office to discuss the results.

"Well, I have some very good news," the doctor said. "You are in tremendous shape. In fact, you've broken a record here at this office. No one else has done this well. You seem like you're the picture of health. Whatever you're doing, just keep it up. It seems to be working for you. Your heart is in great shape."

No heart issues! That was music to my ears, and I let out a loud sigh of relief.

"There's just one thing," the doctor continued. "The only thing I noticed—and it's probably nothing to worry about—is a mole on your lower back. It looks a little different, just a bit suspicious, but it's probably nothing. However, I recommend you have it checked out by a dermatologist the first chance you get." Then he referred me to a dermatologist in the same building.

Immediately my mind went back a few years to when I was twenty-four and my barber had noticed an unusual spot on my head. I had gone to a dermatologist who removed the growth, which turned out to be basal cell carcinoma, a form of skin cancer. After removing it, he told me that I should take precaution in the sun and use plenty of sunscreen. I'd done what he recommended and hadn't given much thought to it since. When I left the doctor that day, I was upset by the fact that the visit had led to yet another doctor's visit—the last thing I wanted or had time for.

On the day of my appointment with the dermatologist, I attended the funeral of another family member. This one was for my granny, my birth mother's mother and the best grandmother anyone could ever wish for. I was so tired of having to say good-bye to the people I loved. After leaving the cemetery, I headed off to my appointment. I waited dutifully, first in the waiting room and then the exam room. And just like before, the nurse told me to take off my shirt, sit on the exam table, and that the doctor would be in shortly.

"What seems to be the problem?" the doctor asked me as he walked in and opened my file.

"I have a mole on my back," I began. "When I was having a cardiac stress test, the doctor noticed it and thought I ought to have it checked out."

"Well," he said, "let's have a look at it."

He walked behind me, paused for a minute or two and then blurted out, "Oh my! I think you might have melanoma!" Now I didn't know much about melanoma at the time. I'd heard of the word, and it sure didn't sound like a friendly word to me. I remember as a child, my stepmother telling me that people could get cancer from moles and that it sometimes killed them. I really couldn't imagine something like that. But the way this doctor was reacting absolutely put the fear of God into me. Almost giddy while examining the mole on my back and without any testing whatso-ever, this dermatologist had jumped to the conclusion it was melanoma. What was worse, he sounded as though he just had discovered the Holy Grail and could not contain his excitement. Maybe this was his first time coming in contact with this sort of thing, I'm not sure, but he went on and on, saying that this was *very* serious and needed to be removed *immedi-ately* and he might have to remove a large portion of tissue from my back as well.

I found his attitude so alarming and uncalled for that I had to get out of there. I mumbled something about, "I'll get back to you." Then I quickly dressed, left his office, and never returned. I had never been so frightened in my life. But I knew one thing for sure. I was not going to let this cancer-happy doctor get a hold of me again. Discovering a potential melanoma may have been exciting to him, but it sure wasn't exciting to me.

My perfect world—my wife, our baby daughter, our home, and the businesses we had built, everything that I was looking forward to in life—came to a sudden and painful halt. Once again, I felt like I had hit a brick wall. If that doctor was right, and I hoped with all my being that he wasn't, my whole world was about to crumble before my eyes.

It's a miracle that I made it home after that appointment as I could barely concentrate on driving. I was in shock. When I shared the news with Mellisa, confessing how upset I was over the possibility of having melanoma, she tried to put my mind at ease. She told me to try not to worry—that it would probably be ok. She also suggested that I get a second opinion right away. That made good sense to me.

First thing the next day, I called and made an appointment with the same dermatologist in Houston who had helped me with the skin cancer on my head all those years ago. He was a nice guy as I remembered and, unlike the previous doctor, had a good bedside manner. I began recalling his words to me back then, "We'll have to keep an eye on things. And don't forget to use sunscreen every day, no matter what. There's a good chance you may get skin cancer again."

After what seemed like years, the day of my appointment finally arrived. The doctor said he remembered me, pulled out my records, and began his examination. I relaxed a little.

"Well," he began in a soothing voice. "It looks kinda' suspicious to me, too. My wife had a stage I melanoma. She had it removed and never had a problem again. This might be something . . . and it might not. I wouldn't worry too much about it. If it is anything serious, it's probably in the early stages. But I think you should have it checked out by someone who specializes in this type of thing. I have a friend here in Houston, Dr. Jones, who is one of the world's best in dealing with this type of thing. I'd like to refer you to him." His nurse made an appointment for me and within a couple of days I found myself in the renowned oncologist's office in downtown Houston.

Dr. Jones also had a decent bedside manner, which I very much appreciated. That sort of thing was becoming more and more important to me. People trust their lives to those wearing white coats. Is it too much to ask that they not scare a guy half to death and maybe even give him a little hope along the way? Dr. Jones looked at the mole on my lower back and said, "It looks a little suspicious to me, too. The only way we'll know what we're dealing with is to remove it and have it tested."

This made perfect sense to me! Enough with all the guessing, let's just find out what we're dealing with. After numbing the area, the doctor removed a sizeable plug from the lower part of my back. He dug deep to get all the surrounding tissue for testing, then sewed me back up and bandaged the area. "I'll send this to the lab for testing and I'll give you a call in the next few days with the results," he said. "There's nothing else to do right now. Just go home and go about your business . . . and don't worry."

Now, I don't know if you've ever been told by a doctor not to worry, but as a patient, that's about the hardest thing you can do, especially if you think you might have something serious. The very thing that you're told not to focus on is the *only* thing you can think about. A few days of waiting for that promised phone call turned into almost two weeks. I paced the floor, couldn't sleep well, and was consumed with worry about the final verdict. I couldn't concentrate on much of anything except that call. Finally, the phone rang and it was the oncologist on the other end. It felt like I had waited years for this call.

"James, this is Dr. Jones. I got your results back from the lab. First, I like to tell you that I have some good news and some bad news," he began. You can pretty much guess the gist of the call will be bad news when someone starts the conversation like this. And, sure enough, it was.

"The good news," he began, "is that it is melanoma."

"The *good news*?" I thought to myself. "How can that be good news?"

"But," Dr. Jones continued, "we think we've got it all. We couldn't find any melanoma around the incision area. That means, hopefully, it hasn't spread outside the tissue we removed from your lower back. That's a good thing."

Then he paused. I held my breath.

"The bad news," Dr. Jones continued, "is that it was very deep. Very deep means that this is stage IV melanoma cancer." My world came to a sudden halt as time seemed to stand still. Then he said something about a scale that measured the different depths, but I was having a hard time concentrating at that point.

"Would you repeat that?" I asked.

"According to the Clark Scale, it is stage IV. That means it is more likely to spread into other parts of the body. We really need to keep a close eye on this. You should come in to see me every three months, and we'll check everything out. There's nothing else you can do. Chances are, we'll never see it again," he added. "Bottom line," he said, "just go live your life and don't worry."

Don't worry? Was he kidding? I was beyond upset now. I had just been told I had stage IV melanoma, which meant (in my mind and from what I knew) that there was a good chance it was going to spread. And the more I thought about it, the worse it seemed to get. Surely this was a bad dream and I would wake up. But it wasn't a dream. It was my new reality.

"You're going to be fine," Mellisa said, trying to comfort me. "You have to quit worrying about it so much. I think it's going to be okay." But the truth was that I couldn't quit worrying about it. It was all I thought about. I felt very alone and sorry for myself. I even felt embarrassed. Here I was, thinking I was the picture of health, running around town, and now I have stage IV cancer. I just wanted to crawl into a hole. The more I read and learned about melanoma, especially the advanced stage, the more fearful I became. Real or not, I began to feel like folks in town were just waiting for me to die.

For me, the three months I had to wait until my next checkup was incredibly stressful. But the three months eventually passed and there I was back in the doctor's office to see how things were progressing. He asked me how I was doing, and all I could say was, "Terrible!"

"Let's see if you really have anything to worry about," he said. First, he looked at the area where the growth had been removed. Next, he felt under my arms and then around my groin area to check my lymph nodes. After the examination, he said, "Everything looks okay. Go on home and we'll see you in three more months." For just a few minutes, hearing what he just told me, I was speechless. These were the very words I was hoping to hear. All I could muster was a simple, "Thank you, Doc."

As time went on, I sometimes felt better. Some days I even began to believe that maybe it would be okay after all. Then I'd start to think about my condition, the words I had read about a diagnosis of melanoma, and I would fall back into depression. Once again, nothing could console me. The fear returned. Where I once was the life of the party, I was no longer fun to be around.

To top it all off, my ambition took a nosedive. I lost interest in managing our businesses. "What was the use, anyway?" I thought. Mellisa stepped up to handle even more of the business chores. Some days, she would leave the baby at home with me while she went to the office, often putting in long hours. It was a lot for her to handle, but I was too wrapped up in my own self-pity to think about what it was doing to her. I'd look at our beautiful daughter and sometimes couldn't hold back the tears, thinking I might not get to see her grow up. I wanted to experience all the milestones in her life. I knew what it was like to lose a parent, and the last thing I wanted was for Carol to have to go through that pain.

As I considered the possibility of my life being cut short, I began to think of all the things I would be missing. Maybe I should make use of the time I had and start doing some of the things I've wanted to do—a bucket list of sorts. I'd always loved Colorado and enjoyed our ski trips there. We had purchased a ski house in Breckenridge where we would sometimes vacation. The longer I thought about it, the more I felt I'd like to live there. I didn't want to die without accomplishing at least some of my dreams. And maybe by leaving Huntsville and starting over, things could change for the better. A new adventure might help to get my mind off my troubles.

My wife, on the other hand, had no desire to pack up everything and move to Colorado and give up everything we had worked so hard to build in Huntsville. My feeling was that she was becoming increasingly impatient with my depressed behavior and I can't say that I blamed her. I was not the same happy-go-lucky person she had married. Instead, I felt like I was dying on the inside. Unless you're the one going through something like this, I realize it's hard to understand. I began to notice a growing distance between us, but I told myself that it was probably normal for married couples, especially those who were working as much as we were and not making marriage a priority. But now that I was distracted with my own illness and watching my life come to an end, I no longer wanted to go anywhere or do much of anything. I was no fun to be around, that's for sure.

One day it all came to a head. My wife told me she had decided to take our daughter and move out. "I'll get an apartment in town and you can stay here in our house. It'll be better that way," she said. I was devastated. I hadn't stopped to consider the toll that my illness and my depression were taking on her. I guess the responsibility of holding things together was just too overwhelming, and she couldn't deal with it any longer. The nicer, fun-loving guy she had married was no longer there. And with the cancer diagnosis, I had changed from someone with ambition, to someone who didn't have the same drive to succeed. All I wanted to do was stay alive! Still, while her decision couldn't have been an easy one for her, it came as a huge blow to me. But I was too wrapped up in my own despair to figure out how to keep her and save our marriage. After she moved out, I didn't care if I lived or died. My once successful life had come to an end. I couldn't help wondering, why me? Why now?

For me, the escape path to easing the emotional pain of being sick, alone, and depressed was simple. Rather than sitting by myself day and night in my house, I started drinking to forget about all my troubles. It had eased the pain after my father's death, so why not now? I started hanging out in bars on the outskirts of town, as I didn't want people in town to see me. I'd play shuffleboard with whoever was there and have a good ol' time, or as much as I could under the circumstances. When you're drinking, everything's okay, until the next day when you wake up and the bad dream is still there.

One day, opportunity came knocking at my door, and I'm so glad I answered! My good friend Bill was involved in a business refurbishing foreclosed homes for home-mortgage companies, and was looking to expand to the Dallas area. He asked if I'd be interested in helping him and his partners get a branch going there. Even in the depressed state I was in, I guess Bill appreciated my aptitude for business. He also thought it might help me if I moved away from Huntsville and had something else to occupy my mind. It turned out to be just what I needed. With little to keep me in Huntsville, I moved to Dallas. I was still close enough to Huntsville that I could visit my daughter regularly.

Bill and his partners put me in charge of the Dallas office. The new position and the challenges it provided gave me a new outlook and focus, which I sorely needed. I had a secretary and a half dozen guys working for me, as well as a variety of contractors who did everything from cleaning, painting, and carpeting to roofing and landscaping. My job was to inspect the houses, assess what repairs were needed, and then create a bid and present it to the mortgage company. If approved, I would then direct my crew to make the needed repairs for each property. We would maintain the properties until they were sold.

I liked the new opportunity and was even beginning to enjoy myself again. I was good at this type of work because of my upbringing and following my father's meticulous way of doing things. And the business was booming! Some days, I'd drive three hundred miles, inspecting different homes. My ambition started kicking in again, and I began thinking about the possibilities of spin-off businesses. The job was good for me in many ways. My friend had been right. It helped to get my mind off the cancer.

I continued going back for my three-month checkups with Dr. Jones, and with each new "all clear" pronouncement, thoughts of my initial diagnosis of cancer began to fade. More and more, I began to think that maybe the cancer really would go away. But what goes up must come down, and just like a roller coaster, I soon hit another bottom. One morning in the shower I felt a lump in my groin. It felt like a small marble. "Oh my God!" I thought as a fresh wave of fear swept through me. It was obviously a new, unwelcome lump. I finished showering and called Dr. Jones in Houston. He said, "Come on down and we'll get you checked out." I wasted no time in flying there.

After he examined me, he said, "Well, I *think* it's okay. Don't worry about it this time. Come back in three months and we'll see how it's doing." Relieved, I went back to Dallas and soon got back into the groove of working. But a short time later, I noticed that the lump was growing. It was unmistakably getting larger. I flew to Houston to see Dr. Jones again, but this time he didn't tell me to go back home and keep a check on it. Instead, he said, "I think we'd better go in and see what this is. Hopefully, it won't be anything. Come on back in the morning and we'll get you checked into the hospital."

That night, I hung out with friends. They were playing volleyball in a league game and having fun. I knew they were trying to cheer me up, but it just wasn't working. It's an awful feeling to be around others when they're happy and having a good time, and all you can think about is that you're going to the hospital the next morning with the possibility of another cancer diagnosis.

Morning came quickly and I checked into a hospital in Houston. It was the first time I had ever had surgery, so the whole experience was new to me. I remember the anesthesiologist talking to me and the next thing I knew the surgery was over and I was in the recovery room. I was groggy when I came to. I could feel a lot of bandages and pressure on my groin. Common sense told me a tiny incision wouldn't require all those bandages. Uh oh. My heart sank. I knew instinctively that something was very wrong. This couldn't be good news.

Dr. Jones soon came in and seeing that I was awake began to tell me what they had found. "Well, I'm sorry to tell you that the cancer has spread to your lymphatic system. We went ahead and removed all the lymph nodes in that area. This is what we were afraid of. It's certainly not the best outcome we were hoping for." My head was spinning as the familiar downward spiraling began. "This sort of cancer spreads fairly rapidly," he continued, "so we're going to have to get going on treating this if we have any chance at all of beating it." I struggled to concentrate on his words in my post-recovery state.

"This particular treatment you'll be getting is experimental. It's about the only thing we've had any measure of success with, so I am recommending it in your case. We're going to do hyperthermia treatments along with chemotherapy. A total of eighty treatments."

"*Eighty* experimental treatments?" I thought to myself. Did I understand that correctly or was this a nightmare? Dr. Jones continued to explain what the treatment involved. It was the most advanced experimental treatment that conventional medicine had to offer for my kind of cancer. "We will elevate your temperature with a hyperthermia serum, a type of typhoid, which we will inject into your veins through an IV drip. The serum will help to stimulate your immune system by inducing a fever to fight the typhoid. The idea is that certain immune cells will be stimulated to become more active for the next few hours and raise the levels of cancer cell-killing compounds in the blood. Then when your immune system is activated, we will induce chemotherapy to fight off the cancer. Heating cancer cells to temperatures above normal makes them easier to destroy with chemotherapy. But careful temperature control is a must with any type of hyperthermia, and so we will be monitoring your temperature carefully."

Dr. Jones continued to inform me of the potential side effects of the proposed treatment. "When we elevate your temperature with the hyperthermia serum, it's going to make you feel like you have a bad case of the flu. Whole-body and regional hyperthermia can cause nausea, vomiting, and diarrhea. More serious, though rare, side effects can include problems with the heart, blood vessels, and other major organs."

He paused as I lay there helplessly in disbelief. "Also," he added, "you will need to regularly use a lymph drainage pump on your leg because of the large number of lymph nodes we had to remove. You must keep your leg elevated when you use the leg pump. If you don't, there is the possibility that you could lose your leg. This is going to take quite a bit of your time, but it can't be ignored. We'll get you a pump so that you can get started on this immediately." A possibility *I could lose my leg*? The nightmare was getting worse by the minute.

"It will take some time to get over the surgery you've just had," he continued. "It will probably be two to three weeks until you can even get around very well. We'll just keep you here in the hospital while you recover. Then when we feel you're up to it, we'll give you the first round of hyperthermia and chemotherapy on the final week. I'll be checking back with you regularly to see how you're doing."

Well, that sounded like a hell of a deal. His recommended treatment was for me to hang around here in the hospital for a couple of weeks, doing all I could to keep from losing my leg after having an unplanned, unexpected number of lymph nodes removed from my groin. Then after I get to feeling good enough, I'd get to start on the first of *eighty* experimental treatments that might or might not work to get rid of the cancer that had now become my worst enemy.

The doctor left me alone to deal with my pain. And pain there was. I wasn't sure which was worse—the emotional pain or the physical. At first, I refused to take any pain meds. I wanted to be a tough guy. But one of the nurses at the hospital gently explained to me that it would be better not to submit my body to such constant pain. Eventually, I gave in and took what they gave me. I had never had morphine before, but it sure did the trick. Within a few minutes, the shot of morphine in my rear made all the pain go away. I could relax and, all of a sudden, things didn't seem so bad. The morphine numbed not only my pain, but also my emotions and made me forget about my troubles . . . until it started to wear off, that is.

I was still very sore and swollen in the groin and upper leg area where the lymph nodes had been removed. I had a ten-inch incision and lots of staples. My entire lower body ached. A tube had been inserted to drain the lymph from that area. Like it or not, and despite the pain, I was told that I had to get up and walk, at least to the bathroom. If I didn't, they would have to insert a catheter. I wanted to avoid that at all costs, so I somehow managed to push through the pain.

Dr. Jones came in every day or so to check on me as promised. Finally, one day I asked him, "Doctor, exactly what are my chances? I know you told me that this cancer has spread into my lymphatic system and that I need the hyperthermia and chemotherapy treatments, but I'd like to know just what my chances are."

"Well," he said, pausing. "I'll be honest with you. I'm sorry to say that you probably have only about a twenty-percent chance of surviving three to five years . . . and that's *if* you can make it through all the chemo treatments. Unfortunately, it's really the best we have to offer. It's a tough go with this stuff, no doubt about it. The key is whether your body will respond to the therapy in a positive way."

"What if I don't do the treatments?" I asked.

"Then I don't think you'll have much more time. The chance of long-term survival isn't great with this therapy, mind you, but I believe it's your best, and practically speaking, only real option.

My only real option.

The words echoed in my mind all through the night.

3

Three Knocks at My Door

*"At any given moment, you have the power to say
this is not how my story is going to end."*
—Anonymous

As I lay in that hospital bed, the thoughts rushing through my head seemed only to add to my stress. I wondered if my grandfather and my daddy had been better off dying quickly instead of suffering each day not knowing when the end would come. There I was in a hospital room alone. I felt like I was just a number, a problem to be fixed on the world's slowest moving assembly line, or worse yet, an experiment in which the outcome is anybody's guess.

I was only thirty-two years old and felt as though I had nothing to live for. My health was in shambles and my wife had taken our baby daughter and left. I had hit a wall and it looked as though I was down for the count. Lying there in my hospital bed, I was feeling miserable and sorry for myself when the phone rang.

"Hello, this is Ron."

Ron was the preacher at the church I sometimes attended back in Huntsville. He was an ex-professional baseball player, a runner, and a tough guy. He also had a streak of kindness that ran deep.

"I just heard about you and your condition," he continued. "I want you to know that I'm praying for you and others are, too. I just want you to know that if anybody can beat this thing, *you* can. Don't you ever forget that."

"Ah, thanks, Ron," I said, probably not sounding like I was buying it.

"No, I mean it," he continued. "Don't give into this. You get in there and you fight! You go out there and you beat this *son-of-a-bitch cancer*."

I was shocked. My preacher was on the phone talking like this? It reminded me of a coach who's giving a pep talk to the losing team at halftime during the championship game. I thought about that conversation long after the phone call ended. He didn't recite one of those prissy, well-rehearsed prayers like some folks would have done. But at that moment, I truly felt the presence of God, the Creator, the Spirit—however you want to define it. Something I really hadn't thought could happen, *happened*. I didn't feel alone anymore.

I realized I was backed into a corner and needed help. I was fighting for my life and unsure what to do next. At that moment, I started doing something I hadn't done for a long time. I prayed. "God, I'm not the best guy in the world. I've done things I'm not proud of. I'm in desperate need of You right now. If you're the God that people say you are, I'm asking for your help. I doubted you, wondering how all this could happen to me—I think I'm a good person. I've asked You for help before, but now I'm asking one hundred times stronger than I've ever asked. I don't know what else to do or who else to go to."

The First Knock at the Door

Praying that intense prayer was quite an experience. I felt like every cell in my body was involved and asking for help. A deep unbelievable sense of calmness came over me. It was like nothing I had ever felt before, and I began to relax. No more than twenty minutes later, I heard a knock on the door.

Ronnie Davidge, a college friend of mine who I hadn't seen in over seven years, came through the door with some papers in his hand. "I heard about you from one of our old friends," he said. "He told me you were in the hospital . . . and battling cancer." Ronnie had wanted to come visit me, but wasn't sure when it would be the right time. But on that very day he was driving around the area and had a strong feeling that *now* was the time.

"It's like this," Ronnie continued. "I was talking to someone at lunch the other day, and he told me about an article he had read about a guy who cured himself of cancer using a special diet. He said he thought maybe you'd be interested in it, so he brought me the article to give to you." I felt an excitement stir deep within my body. Somehow I just *knew* this was an answer to my prayer! As he handed the article to me, I looked him in the eye and said, "This is what I am going to do. This is my ticket to getting well." I probably sounded like a crazy person, but that was the way I felt.

Ronnie chuckled, "Wait a minute, you haven't even read it yet! You don't know anything about it. How can you be so sure?"

"I don't have to read it," I said. "I just know this is what I'm supposed to do." I opened the pages he had given me and began to read. It was a copy of a book review in *Let's Live* magazine about the healing journey of actor Dirk Benedict. Benedict had starred as Lieutenant Starbuck in the original *Battlestar Galactica* movie and television series. He also played Lieutenant Templeton "Face" Peck in *The A-Team* TV series, which I had seen many times. "Hmmm," I smiled. I had never realized his character's first name was Templeton, the same as mine. Maybe I was grasping at straws, but if that wasn't a sign, what was?

The article mentioned that the actor, who had been raised on a ranch in Montana, found himself with all the symptoms of prostate cancer when he was in his thirties. But instead of submitting to the standard chemotherapy treatments, he found a way to heal himself with a special diet—the macrobiotic diet. I had never heard of such a thing, but I knew in my heart it was going to be the key to my healing.

Where I come from, when you get sick, you go to a doctor. You don't go on a new diet. But the idea was new and very exciting to me. The book review inspired me so much, I must have read it ten times. I looked up at Ronnie and thanked him for the article. Then I asked him for a favor. Could he please get me a copy of Dirk's book, *Confessions of a Kamikaze Cowboy*? He dropped off the book the very next day. That was the last time I saw my friend.

As I began reading the book, I became more and more inspired. The pain in my body was still there, but I was so excited over what I was reading that I didn't notice it as much. It sounded cool to me. Dirk had driven around the country on what was a healing journey. The macrobiotic diet he followed had him eating lots of whole grains, fresh vegetables (sometimes he ate fresh corn right from the fields), and something called miso soup. It sounded like a journey of true healing. That's what I wanted. I didn't want to do what everyone else was doing, especially after being told that I had very little chance of survival on their prescribed treatments. What kind of outlook was that? And just like Dirk, I wanted to be the hero in my own life and find something to give me hope and a chance to go on living. I could relate to this guy and his big spread in Montana. After all,

I was a Texan and had my own spread. My whole outlook and sense of well-being changed after reading Dirk's story. "If he can do it," I thought, "I can, too!"

I knew the inspiration had come from a higher power. It gave me a new strength and the positive outlook I badly needed. Now I had *hope.* And hope was the key to everything at that point in my life. I was going to hold onto that hope tighter than I had ever held onto anything before.

The Second Knock at the Door

The next day, there was another knock on the door. It was Mama. She had a book in her hand, *Vitamin C and Cancer* by Dr. Linus Pauling. "I thought you might be interested in this," she said as she handed me the book. I immediately read the copy on the back cover to see what it was about. Dr. Pauling was a biochemist and peace activist who won two Nobel Prizes—the first in chemistry in 1954, followed by a Nobel Peace Prize in 1962. Over the years, he had studied the health effects of vitamin C. His research had shown that people who took high amounts of the vitamin tended to live a lot longer than people who didn't. It also explained how terminally ill cancer patients had been given vitamin C to keep them alive for quite some time. When the vitamin C was stopped, they would die.

"Thanks, Mama." I said. "This is great!" When she left, I began reading and learned about Dr. Pauling's findings. I became more and more excited by all the new things I was learning. What could possibly be the harm in trying vitamin C? What did I have to lose? This surely was another answer to my prayer. Now I had even more hope and an even better chance that I might beat this cancer after all. I felt my fighting spirit returning. "Nothing's going to take my life away from me without a real fight." Then and there I decided that *no way* was I going back to the year of fear that I had just lived through.

The Third Knock at the Door

The next day, there was another knock on the door. "Come in!" I called from my hospital bed. "Good Morning," the stranger said. "I'm the hospital psychotherapist and I'm here to help you. I've heard that you've had a pretty rough time of it recently, and I'd like to talk to you. Would tomorrow be a good time for me to come back and visit?" I had several visitors come by to see me in the hospital, but I knew the last two had definitely brought me important messages. And while I had no idea what this gentleman was going to tell me, whatever it was, I was willing to listen. "Tomorrow's fine," I quickly said.

By the time he came back the next day, I had been doing a lot of reading—and thinking—about the macrobiotic diet. So as soon as he walked over to my bed, I said, "Hey, before we get started, I wanted to ask if you've ever heard of some diet called macrobiotic?" He looked at me, hesitated, and then said, "Hold on a second." He went over to the door, which was ajar, and closed it quietly, but firmly. Then he pulled up a chair and sat down next to my bed.

"First of all, I would love to tell you what I know about the macrobiotic diet, but this has to be confidential," he began. "You have to promise not to tell anyone that we've ever spoken about this. I've been working here a long time, and I don't want to lose my job, my benefits, or my pension. The people who run this oncology floor are not going to be happy with me if I talk to you about this. Will you promise me?"

Right at that moment, I knew that if he knew something about this diet and didn't want anyone to know that he's telling me about it, then I *really* must be onto something. He went on to tell me that he knew quite a bit about the macrobiotic diet and lifestyle. He had heard a lot of good things about the diet and there were many success stories of critically ill cancer patients using the diet with great success. "But," he cautioned. "It's not easy. It takes a lot of time and energy. It's a full-time job. You have to roll up your sleeves and do whatever it takes." Seeing that his words didn't faze me, he continued. "You'll have to read everything you can about the macrobiotic diet. You'll have to learn to cook a certain type of food and prepare it a certain way. It's not for everyone. I tried doing it myself, but it was too hard for me to stick with. It took up too much of my time, but I do think it is a good system for some people." He paused. "The chemotherapy route is a tough go, and the cancer that you have is a very serious one. You can't do this diet halfway," he said again. "You have to really stick with it. If you can do that, I think it could help you a lot. I had heard that you were very depressed, but after talking to you, it seems like you're motivated to do something. I think that this would really be good for someone like you."

He told me about two other books that I should read *Recalled by Life* and *Living Well Naturally,* both by Dr. Anthony J. Sattilaro. I was beyond excited. Now I had *three* answers to my urgent prayer—Dirk Benedict's book, important information about vitamin C, and the positive words of the hospital psychotherapist regarding the macrobiotic diet. And soon I would have two more books in my hands by Dr. Sattilaro.

I knew I was onto something. I was determined to be the next guy telling my healing story someday. That's what I felt in my heart that I was supposed to do. God had given me the tools, and now it was up to me to go out and be successful. This was my second chance. Maybe I wouldn't have to leave my little girl fatherless after all. I wasn't going to let God down, I wasn't going to let myself down, and I definitely wasn't going to look back. It was time to look forward. I felt like I had a mission—first to help myself and then to help others.

4

Two O'Clock in the Morning

"Sometimes the smallest step in the right direction ends up being the biggest step of your life. Tip toe if you must, but take a step."
—NAEEM CALLAWAY

Full of hope and armed with a new plan, I was ready to get started with the experimental treatments. I was not about to give in without a fight in my commitment to defeat stage IV melanoma. To my way of thinking, I could combine the recommended treatments with the macrobiotic diet and vitamin C and beat this thing even quicker. Hell, maybe I wouldn't even need all of their treatments.

During the third week of my hospital stay, still recovering from the surgery in which all of my lymph nodes had been removed from my right groin, the men in the white coats decided I was strong enough to begin their prescribed treatments, the best they had to offer. "Mr. Templeton, in the morning, we'll begin the first five-day round of the chemotherapy and experimental hyperthermia treatment," explained the doctor. "Whole-body hyperthermia raises a person's body temperature to create a fever. This helps chemotherapy work better to treat cancer that has metasta-sized. We're hoping your body will respond positively to the treatments, of course, but we won't know until we try."

Bright and early the next morning, they hooked an IV into a vein on the back of my left hand where first the typhoid serum and later the chemo would be injected. The purpose of the typhoid serum was to stim-ulate my immune system by raising my body temperature until it was between 104° and 105°F. It was important that it didn't go over 105°, as that would be dangerous. Then they placed a "cooling cap" on my head. It was supposed to help keep my hair from falling out from the chemo. I think it would be more appropriate to call it an ice cap, as it was extremely cold. Lastly, they placed weighted blankets on me. I soon found out why. Shortly after the serum was being released into my system, I began to feel cold all over, but it was a cold like I've never felt before. The chills and fever came fast, robbing me of my strength.

I was absolutely freezing as I lay there. I'd had the flu before and I'd had fevers, but nothing in the world prepared me for how I felt during this treatment. It was ten times worse than any flu I'd ever suffered. I was shaking uncontrollably and felt like I was in a freezer. It reminded me of a dog in the wintertime that's shaking from the cold. To this day, every time I see a dog shaking in the freezing snow, I think of myself back in that bed.

The typhoid drip took an hour or so to administer. When it was complete, the nurses swapped it out for the chemotherapy drip. All in all, the treatment lasted nearly ten hours. I lay there all day in the worse agony I had ever known. Plus, I was still sore from the lymph-node surgery. I felt like I had been gutted, and I was sporting a ten-inch incision complete with stitches. That, along with the nearly unbearable cold and fever of this new treatment was excruciating. I'd never felt so bad.

When the treatment was finally over, they brought me food. I was able to eat a little that day, but in the days that followed, I was so nauseous I couldn't eat a bite. Through sheer grit, I made it through the five days of treatment. Determined to beat this cancer, I was willing to go to hell and back if I had to—and it felt like I already had. After the last treatment that week, I was released from the hospital. I could barely walk around or fend for myself, so with Mellisa gone, I went to my stepmother's house to recover. Even though I felt awful, I was determined to start the macrobiotic diet. I quickly realized it was going to take a lot of effort to cook and keep up with this diet, as the hospital psychotherapist had warned me. Thank God Mama was there to help.

"What can I do?" Mama asked me. The first thing I needed was a macrobiotic cookbook, and she picked up a couple for me. We would look through them, find a recipe, and then go to the grocery store to look for the ingredients. There was a small health food store in our town, but it didn't carry most of the items I needed. Mama and I did the best we could with what we could find.

Things had greatly changed since my days of being a runner. While I was recovering from that first round of treatments, every day I tried to walk as much as I possibly could. At first, I could only make it from the front door of the house to the gate and back. Gradually, I built up my strength, and was able to walk down the highway a little further each day. I had to drain the lymph from my leg every day and every night. I followed the instructions religiously, as I had no desire to lose my leg. I've since learned that the build-up of lymph, called *lymphedema* is cancer's dirty little secret—a little-known side effect with a huge impact on those of us who have had lymph nodes removed. In the daytime, I would lie in bed with my leg propped up on a pillow while using the pump. I'd pass the time by reading about the macrobiotic lifestyle. I learned to sleep with the leg pump at night. After a couple of weeks of recovery at Mama's house, I was able to go back to work in Dallas. After all, I still needed to earn a living. And it would be a couple of months before my next treatment.

Thank God I had some great people working with me. Though I had been managing the location in Dallas, everyone there at the office had pitched in and kept things running in my absence. They were very supportive, and I was enormously grateful. I realize more and more as life goes on that you're only as good as the help you have. Everyone pitched in as a team and picked up the slack when I couldn't. I felt so bad at first, that sometimes I would have to lay my head on my desk just to get my energy back before starting another task. Little by little though, I gained strength.

Every day I had to cook for myself. I lived in an apartment that had an electric stove, which is a "no-no" for macrobiotic cooking. So I bought a Coleman camp stove and a pressure cooker, which I set on the kitchen counter. It wasn't ideal, but it was the best I could do. I bought organic food from the Whole Foods Market in Dallas.

According to the macrobiotic lifestyle, each mouthful of food should be chewed at least 50 times before swallowing. I decided if that was good, I'd do even better and chew each mouthful 180 times. As you might guess, mealtimes took awhile. I would get up at 4:30 in the morning and put my breakfast on before going out for a walk, which still caused pain in my leg. Little by little, I got stronger and stronger. Eventually, I worked up to two miles, although I would be stiff and sore afterwards. Before I left for my walks, as recommended in my cookbooks, I would put brown rice in the pressure cooker, then place it on the camp stove over a very low flame (with a flame tamer). By the time I got back from my walks, which took forty-five minutes or more, my brown rice breakfast would be ready, and I would have it with some miso soup. After breakfast, I'd grab leftovers from last night's dinner for my lunch, and then head out to be at work by seven.

Little by little, I began to add more to my daily routine. Through my reading, I learned about a stretching exercise called Dōln, which, along with stretching, involves tapping on the different meridians of the body to keep the energy flowing correctly. I found it to be very helpful. I was determined not to cut any corners. The hospital psychotherapist's words about the macrobiotic diet were embedded in my memory—the people who do it right get the best results. The more I learned—and I read every chance I got—the more determined I became. One recommendation of the macrobiotic lifestyle is to never go to bed sooner than three hours after eating. This is so all the body's energy at night can be directed toward healing, not digestion. If I got through eating dinner at seven or eight, I wouldn't lie down for at least three hours, even if it meant sitting in a chair to read or meditate. I also tried visualization techniques. I'd visualize myself completely healthy and pain free. Sometimes I'd be so tired I'd nearly fall asleep, but never would I go to bed within that three-hour time frame.

And always, always I would use the leg pump. On weekends, I'd be able to use it during the daytime, but with my long hours at work on weekdays, there was no way. So I continued to sleep with it every night. I was still having a hard time with walking. My leg would often swell and my groin was still very painful. One night I got to thinking about it. "I can't run, I can barely walk. But I bet I could ride a bicycle!" So the next day I bought a ten-speed bike.

Every day after work, even though it was late, I would ride my bike around White Rock Lake in Dallas. The path around the lake was a little over two-and-a-half miles and I would go around a few times every evening or as much as I could. When it came to bike-riding, the hardest part was getting my leg over the cross bar. And with my sore groin, sitting on the bike wasn't exactly a piece of cake. But I bought a more comfortable seat, which made it a lot better. I always worried about getting into a bike wreck, but, thankfully, never did. Each day I got stronger and eventually worked up to bicycling a hundred miles a week.

It had taken me a few weeks to get in the groove and figure things out according to the macrobiotic way. I was beginning to get a handle on it. And it had taken me two months to get over feeling nauseous from the treatments I had in the hospital. Finally, I was starting to feel like something positive was changing in my body. By then, however, it was time for another round of treatments—another week in the hospital in Houston.

While waiting at the hospital to be admitted, I remember talking with other cancer patients who were also scheduled for treatments. "Yeah, I'm going in to get my chemo," one guy said to me. "This is hopefully my last bout for awhile. How long are you in here for?" Another particularly nice woman remarked, "I can't wait to get my chemo and get back to normal life again." When my room was ready, I wished the other patients well, and then waited for the torture to begin. Once the session began, I wondered if they had doubled or tripled my doses because this round was so bad that it made the first round seem like a cake walk. I had never been so sick in my life.

In planning for the week's hospital stay, I had asked Mama and one of my friends to please pick up prepared food for me from the local macrobiotic center in Houston. Since I obviously couldn't cook for myself while in the hospital, I wanted to do the best I could to stay on the diet. They picked up meals for me as planned, but I was so sick, I couldn't eat much after the first day or two.

I remember lying in the hospital bed after the daily treatments were over. Every night, Catholic nuns would visit the patients. I was so drugged up with morphine that I began hallucinating. Sometimes I would see the nuns "float" through my room in their white habits and think angels were visiting me. It felt like a sign of peace. Other times, in my hallucinatory state, I would think the drugs that had been injected into my veins were from the devil and were going to kill me, not help me.

Each day, the doctor would stop in and ask, "How are you doing?"

"I feel like hell, I'm sick, and I can't eat," I'd tell him. "This can't be good!"

He'd say, "Well, unfortunately, your body is not responding very well. But let's just keep after it and, hopefully, your body will accept the chemo."

Often at night, I would hear other patients down the hallway moaning and groaning. At times, the whole floor sounded like a torture chamber. But I was so sick, all I could do was lie there, wishing the madness would stop. Occasionally, there would be a commotion on the floor, and I'd ask the nuns, "What's happening out there?" "Well, so-and-so passed away," they'd answer. One time, they mentioned the name of the woman I had spoken with in the admitting area just a couple days earlier, the one who was looking forward to the chemo treatments so that she could get back to a normal life. She had lost her battle with cancer. How in the world could she die in just a few short days? I learned that many of the patients were dying of pneumonia and other illnesses. Their immune systems must have been trashed from the chemotherapy. I began to wonder if I'd be lucky enough to get out of there alive.

One particularly rough day that week, all I could do was lie in bed, feeling like I was dying inside. I probably was. I was getting weaker and weaker each day, and that day was the absolute worst. If someone had come in with a gun, I would have told them to shoot me . . . or give me the gun and I'd do it myself. Realizing I felt that bad really scared me. I was hanging on by a thread. I began to realize that staying in this hospital was taking away my hope and everything I was fighting for. When a nurse came in, I could barely come out of my drugged-up stupor and open my eyes to see her. "Oh my God!" I heard her say. "Who's been watching over this man? His temperature is way, *way* too high! We have to get it down *now!*" Several hospital staff came rushing in and started putting cold wet towels on me, trying to cool me down. Apparently, they hadn't been keeping a close eye on my elevated temperature. No wonder I felt so bad!

When I started feeling a little more alive, I made up my mind to get out of that damn hospital before it was too late. I decided when the doctor came in, I was going to have a heart-to-heart talk with him. When he finally came around, he said, "I hear you've been having a hard time with your treatments?"

"Yeah," I said. "I can't imagine being this sick. I'm not so sure this is the best thing. How can this be good for me?"

"Well, I hate to tell you," he said. "But the results aren't what we hoped for. Your body isn't responding to the treatments, and that's not a good sign. We hoped you would be able to withstand them better."

"There's got to be something else I can do!" I replied. "Surely there is some other alternative treatment, some other way?"

"No," the doctor said. "There's nothing else you can do."

"What would you do if it was your son or daughter in my condition?" I pressed him.

"I'd do the same thing," he said.

"Really? You'd do the same thing? You'd torture them with this treatment even if they weren't responding?" I asked him. "What about a natural diet or vitamin C therapy? Are you sure there isn't anything else I can do?"

"No, none of that works," he said. "It's a waste of time."

"Doctor, I don't want the *treatment* to kill me! That's no way to die!" I said.

"Well . . . *we're all going to die someday,*" he replied. I was amazed, shocked that he would say such a thing in such a casual way. His words hit me hard and really made me mad. I couldn't believe how callous he was. I felt like a guinea pig in a failed experiment. I did everything I could to sit up in that hospital bed and said, "Listen here you son of a bitch. If I could get out of this bed, I'd tear you apart!" He turned as white as a ghost and ran out the door. He knew I meant it. That was the last time I saw that doctor.

After he left, I lay there and thought about what he'd said. He could offer nothing more than the experimental treatments, which he admitted weren't working. Yet, I was reading and learning about alternative cancer treatments that had worked for others. If they could work for others, why wouldn't they work for me? I'd never know unless I tried. And what did I have to lose? All I knew was that I couldn't spend one more day in that hospital, so I made a plan. It was "do or die." Literally. That decision turned out to be the most critical fork in the road in my search for health— the first step in my journey to escape a death sentence from cancer.

At two o'clock in the morning, I knew it was time. I struggled to get into my clothes. I was so thin and weak, it took all my strength just to get my jeans on. I felt and looked like a prisoner in a concentration camp. I slowly opened the door to my room and looked out. There was no one in the hallway and it was very quiet. The nurses' station wasn't too far down the hallway and I didn't see anyone sitting there. I slipped out of my room and hobbled down the hall in the opposite direction of the nurses' station. Staying as close as I could to the wall, I eased my way to the stairs, being careful not to make any noise or slam any doors. Somehow, I made it down the stairwell, hanging onto the rails. It took everything I had to make it down those steps. I stumbled out of the hospital into the parking lot and managed to get into my Jeep. I drove to the gate, paid my parking fee, and left . . . never to return. And while it may not have been a dashing escape, it was a successful one.

Mama lived an hour north of the hospital and that's where I headed. I had to stop twice on the interstate just to throw up. There was no question that Mama was surprised to see me, especially at that hour in the morning. "I can't take their treatments anymore," I told her. "I'm going 100-percent macrobiotic." I went straight to bed and slept soundly. The next morning, Mama fixed me some oatmeal. It wasn't the ideal macrobiotic choice, but it was the best she had and I was grateful.

I knew the time had come for me to roll up my sleeves and go to war. I had walked, or in this case, crawled away from conventional medicine, and there was no turning back. Somehow, I had survived. Now it was time for me to take full responsibility for my health. I had to become my own guide, my own doctor, and I wasn't going to look back and feel sorry for myself. I had done enough of that. I made a conscious decision to only look forward. Above all, I was going to hang on to my hope. I was going to put all of my effort into regaining my health through natural means. I would do everything I could down to the letter. "I will not go down easy. I'll go down scratching, clawing, and swinging!" became my battle cry.

After a few days, the nausea from the chemo began to subside, and by eating a healing macrobiotic diet, I began to feel a little more human. I hadn't yet started taking vitamin C but decided now was the time. I didn't know what kind of vitamin C to take or how much, but I bought what they were selling at the local store and made do.

When I got my strength back, I visited my little girl, my Carol, before heading back to Dallas. At that point, I had really dug into my new self-prescribed healing regimen. I knew it wasn't going to be easy, but I didn't care. I was absolutely determined to succeed, come hell or high water. I moved to a different apartment, one with a gas stove. Although the Coleman stove had served me well, it took forever to cook a meal and I had had enough of it. My new apartment was also closer to the Whole Foods Market, another plus. It was just outside the edge of Highland Park, an affluent Dallas neighborhood. The streets were peaceful and made walking a pleasure. The beautiful homes and estates were inspiring and somehow gave me a sense that not only was I going to get well, but I had a future to look forward to again. I began to dream about being healthy and successful, but in a different way than before. I wondered if I could find a way to use my newfound ambition to help others who might be fighting the same fight I was.

But it was a lonely life. Most of my time outside the office was spent shopping at health food stores, cooking, and doing my exercises. There was no one to hang out with except my co-workers, and I didn't go to restaurants since they didn't serve the kind of food I needed. I yearned for like-minded people to share my feelings and my newfound philosophy. It's just human nature to want that, I suppose. And I sure did miss my daughter. But I knew that I had to focus on getting well if I was to be there for her in the long run.

I had read a lot about the Kushi Institute, a macrobiotic teaching center located in the Berkshire Mountains in western Massachusetts. Run by Michio Kushi, it was the leading center for macrobiotic education in the world. I had never been to New England, but I felt I could learn even more about the macrobiotic way if I spent time there. Besides, I needed to meet other people who were living the macrobiotic lifestyle.

It had been over six months since my escape from the hospital and those experimental cancer treatments. I was feeling much better. My heart and lungs were strong, thanks to the running I had done in the past. Looking back now, I think running had helped prepare me for this journey, although I didn't know it back then. I decided it was time to travel to Becket, Massachusetts, to attend one of the Kushi Institute's week-long residential seminars. It turned out to be one of the best weeks of my life.

5

Not All Who Wander
Are Lost

*"I fight for my health every day in ways that
most people don't understand."*
—Anonymous

To my Texas eyes and my lonely spirit, Becket, Massachusetts, was perhaps the most beautiful place on the planet. I didn't know the leaves on trees could be so colorful, so vibrant. No wonder people make pilgrimages to New England in the fall. It had taken about three months for me to really start feeling better after those experimental treatments. I was cooking for myself using all the macrobiotic principles I had learned and was practicing the recommended Dōln exercises as best I could, but I was really looking forward to learning more.

I wanted to seek out macrobiotic experts and learn from them. And I knew the best in the world were at the Kushi Institute. The Institute's founder, Michio Kushi, was the man I really wanted to meet. In *Kamikaze Cowboy*, Dirk Benedict had talked about how he drove across the country to meet Michio. Dirk was also the one who initially got me interested in the macrobiotic diet. I decided to take off a week from work at the Dallas office and signed up for a week-long residential seminar at the Kushi Institute. I had a great team of very capable people working at the office who would cover for me while I was gone—a huge relief.

The Kushi Institute was founded in 1978 by Michio and Aveline Kushi. Michio was regarded by many as the foremost authority on the study and practice of macrobiotics. Born in Japan in 1926, Michio graduated from Tokyo University with a degree in International Law. In 1949, he came to the United States to study governmental law at Columbia University.

Michio had learned about holistic nutrition from George Ohsawa, born Nyoichi Sakurazawa, who is often credited as the founder of the macrobiotic way. Ohsawa taught that eating natural foods, such as whole grains and vegetables, contributed to health and even to world harmony. In his books, Ohsawa explained how he cured himself of tuberculosis at age nineteen by applying the ancient Chinese concept of yin and yang in conjunction with the teachings of Dr. Sagen Ishizuka, a nineteenth-century Japanese doctor. Ohsawa defined health on the basis of seven criteria: lack of fatigue, good appetite, good sleep, good memory, good humor, precision of thought and action, and gratitude.

In the early 1950s, Kushi left New York City along with his wife, Aveline, and their family, and moved to Boston. Over the next few decades, the couple founded a number of health and wellness companies and organizations, including the Kushi Institute, Erewhon Natural Foods, the *East West Journal*, and One Peaceful World Press. A worldwide lecturer, Kushi is credited with introducing macrobiotics to the United States. He wanted to teach people how to eat healthy in order to prevent disease and, he believed, achieve world peace.

At the start of my journey, I flew from Texas to Boston and then took a bus to Lee, Massachusetts, where a staff member from the Institute picked me up. Her name was Susan and she immediately made me feel welcome. After the customary introductions, she asked me why I had come. I didn't feel like going into any details, so all I said was, "I have cancer." My response didn't seem to faze her at all. In fact, I was struck by her casual attitude toward my mentioning the word cancer. She made it seem like cancer was little more than a head cold, something that could be treated easily.

"You've come to the right place. I'm sure you're going to be fine," said my new friend. I felt my spirits begin to lift. It was one thing to read about the successes of the macrobiotic diet and lifestyle, and quite another to be talking face to face with someone who had actually witnessed them at the Institute.

We made our way through the Berkshire Mountains and up a rocky road until we reached the Kushi Institute, which was located at the top of a hill. There were three buildings: the main house, a dormitory, and a large garage. The main house was a beautiful, rustic Tudor mansion made of dark brick with a stone portico above the front door and a terrace that overlooked the front of the house. Originally built as a large hunting lodge, it was now being used as an educational center. The nearby dormitory had once been a monastery. As I got out of the car and looked around, I felt like I had stepped into a Norman Rockwell painting. The sky, the scenery, the house, the little village in the valley below created a beautiful setting—a sight for sore eyes.

It was a cold and beautiful October Sunday afternoon when I walked into the main house for the first time. I took off my shoes just inside the front door as was the custom and set them alongside the numerous pairs of shoes that were already there. I was immediately welcomed by a group of people who invited me to join them in the living room for tea. About twenty-five guests—all from different parts of the world—were there for the seminar. Some, like me, had cancer and were there grasping for hope. Others were dealing with debilitating or chronic illnesses like the Epstein-Barr virus. Some had lost loved ones to various illnesses and were looking for ways to prevent those illnesses in their own lives. Still others were interested in becoming professional macrobiotic chefs and educators. All of us were there to learn from the best of the best.

On the far wall of the living room was a huge and welcoming fireplace. The dining room and kitchen were on the same floor. A large stairway led to the upper floors where the guest sleeping quarters were located and where some of the staff lived. I would be sharing one of the twelve or so bedrooms with another guest who was also there for the seminar. After a pleasant afternoon of getting acquainted with everyone and a brief walk outside in the crisp air, it was time for dinner.

I had been cooking for myself day in and day out for months and let me tell you, that buffet—filled with food that looked and smelled delicious—was a real treat! One side of the buffet featured dishes for those of us with special dietary needs. The other side featured a wider menu for those whose diets weren't quite so strict. The ingredients of all the dishes were listed so we were able to pick and choose as necessary. Students, staff, and visitors all joined together for the meal. We filled our plates and sat down to eat. There were chopsticks, although forks were available for anyone who wanted them. I had never used chopsticks, but I soon learned how. For the next several years, I used them for my meals, and to my surprise, found eating with them to be an almost spiritual experience.

After dinner, we all gathered around the fireplace for orientation. Members of the staff—some of the top macrobiotic educators in the world—told us what to expect during the upcoming week. Listening to them reminded me again how happy I was to be there. Charles Millman and Ed Esko led off the presentation, explaining some of the basics of the macrobiotic way—that it was more than just a diet. It was a lifestyle. They presented a number of lifestyle suggestions that could be naturally integrated into a person's individual life. For example:

- Walk outside in the fresh air two times every day for thirty minutes or longer. In the summertime, it is great to walk barefoot on the grass or on the beach.

- Try to wear 100-percent cotton clothing next to the skin and use cotton sheets and pillowcases on your bed. Cotton allows a smooth flow of energy with the environment. Outer garments and blankets may be of other materials.

- Try to use natural quality body care products and cosmetics. They may be better for personal health as well as for the environment.

- To minimize radiation exposure, limit television or exposure to other artificial electromagnetic fields, preferably to thirty minutes a day. Take regular breaks. For example, if you have to work at a computer all day, get up and stretch at least once an hour.

- Maintain a clean, orderly home and environment.

- Keep green plants in your home and office to increase oxygen and improve air circulation.

- Try to keep active from morning to night. Greet everyone you meet, and maintain active communications with parents, children, and other relatives.

- Light to moderate exercise, including yoga, martial arts, dancing or sports, is also beneficial.

- Self-reflect a few minutes each day on your life and express your appreciation to God, nature, or the universe. This may take the form of prayer, meditation, chanting, and visualization including the creation of healthful, positive thoughts and images.

- Sing a happy song each day!

After the orientation, we all sat around and just talked. It was a very cold evening with snow flurries in the air. I had always loved the cold, though there wasn't much of it where I lived in Texas. So this new climate suited me perfectly. I was so glad to be there. I didn't feel alone any longer. Tired from our travels, we said goodnight to one another and went upstairs. The bedrooms were furnished very sparsely, and we slept on simple futons. I said a prayer of thanks as my head hit the pillow. I slept deeply through the night.

I don't know if you've ever awakened to the smell of fresh whole grains cooking, but let me tell you, it is one of the best things ever. You don't get the same deep aroma with ordinary grains or breakfast from a box. That heavenly smell would permeate the hallways and all the rooms of that big ol' house. My bedroom happened to be above the kitchen, so I really got a good dose of it and looked forward to the silent wake-up call each morning. To this day, I can still remember that wonderful aroma.

Before breakfast, we'd gather in the living room for morning DōIn exercises. We'd lie on the floor and stretch and tap the meridians in our body to get the energy flowing smoothly. DōIn was new to some of my fellow students, but I had been practicing it regularly, so I felt totally at ease. If there was enough time, we'd go outside for a quick walk in the brisk air before breakfast. Breakfast consisted of those wonderful aromatic grains, miso soup, some lightly steamed vegetables, and condiments. To drink, there was hot kukicha tea. Kukicha is a Japanese blend of stems, stalks, and twigs from a type of evergreen shrub (Camellia sinensis) used to make tea. It has a unique flavor and aroma, as it is composed of parts of the plant that are not usually used. The breakfast may have been simple, but it was very delicious and nourishing. Above all, it was healing.

I had been raised on the typical American diet of white bread, meat, milk, eggs, and plenty of fast food. During my running days, just before discovering I had cancer, I had been eating a lot of salads and very little protein. I also drank a lot of milk. Most of my life I had suffered with allergies, which got worse as I got older. Interestingly, after I changed to the macrobiotic diet when I was living in Texas and stopped drinking milk, my allergies completely cleared up. It was one of the first things I experienced that showed me just how much of an impact the food we eat could have on our body.

Learning more about how the macrobiotic diet helps the body achieve and maintain the balance of yin and yang energies—and how all foods have their own natural balance—was an exciting new venture for me. The imbalance of yin or yang can cause ill health, and the right foods are helpful in maintaining a healthy balance. A body with excess heat (yang) needs cooling foods to bring it back into balance. A body with excess cold (yin) needs warming foods. According to the macrobiotic philosophy, foods with a high yang content are warming and energizing. They tend to be salty, bitter, or sour. Meats and salty cheese are examples of yang foods. Foods with more yin content, such as fruit, honey, and vegetables that grow above the ground, are cooling in nature and tend to be sweeter and more neutral.

Coming to terms with my role in how cancer develops was another eye-opener. The real proof that the macrobiotic diet was helping to heal me was in how I felt. Gone were the grueling days of nausea and lack of appetite from the chemotherapy and hyperthermia treatments that nearly killed me. I never felt as high in my life as I did from eating the pure and simple macrobiotic foods. And after exercising on a regular basis, I discovered I didn't have to use the lymph pump as often. I was getting stronger and stronger each day and had never felt more hopeful.

After a short break following breakfast, our first class began. It was on the philosophy of the macrobiotic way, the do's and don'ts. The lecturer began:

The macrobiotic diet is almost like a mix between Buddhism and veganism. The term "macrobiotic" comes from the original Greek meaning of the term "macrobios" or "great life." And again, we learned that yin foods are said to be "passive" and include cold foods and sweets. Yang foods, on the other hand, are more "aggressive" and consist of warm and/or salty foods. A diet should include a balance between yin and yang foods; it should not include too many sweets or too many salty snacks.

A basic tenet of the macrobiotic philosophy is that all things—our bodies, foods, and everything else—are composed of both yin and yang energies. Yin energies are outward moving, yang energies are inward. Everything has both yin and yang energies, with either yin or yang in excess. Most foods that make up the standard American diet have very strong yin or yang properties and also tend to be acid-forming. By contrast, the macrobiotic diet encourages two food groups—grains and vegetables—that have the least pronounced yin and yang qualities. These foods make it easier to achieve a more balanced condition within the natural order of life. Living within the natural order means eating only what is necessary for one's condition and desires. It also means learning to adjust to life's changes in a peaceful way. Learning the effects of different foods allows one to consciously counteract other influences and maintain a dynamically balanced state. The resulting freedom from fear and the new sense of control are two of the most important benefits of a macrobiotic practice.

Handing out two sheets of paper with a chart on each, he continued:

In addition, macrobiotics stresses the use of whole, organic foods grown without pesticides or preservatives. Factors such as where the food was grown, how it was handled, etc., all affect the food's energy, which in turn affects us when we eat it. Nothing should be processed. In addition, it is important to eat foods that are in season and to eat while in a relaxed state of mind. Giving thanks for the nourishment of our food to our bodies is also important.

YIN AND YANG FOOD CHART

This chart presents foods that range from very yin to very yang. As you can see, whole grains, beans, and sea vegetables are those foods with the least pronounced yin and yang qualities. They are the primary foods on the macrobiotic diet.

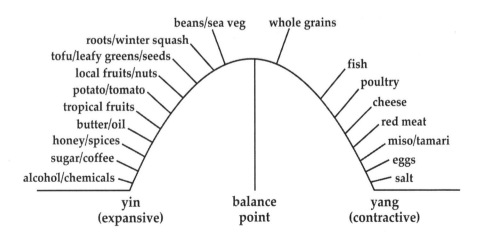

THE GREAT LIFE PYRAMID

This pyramid depicts the principal categories of food that may be taken on a daily or regular basis (five to seven times a week); foods that may be taken weekly or occasionally (one to three times a week) by those in good health; foods that may be consumed monthly or less frequently. The last category, represented by foods at the top of the pyramid, consists of animal quality foods, including meat and dairy, which are not suited to a temperate climate or environment, and may cause health problems. They are included primarily for those in the general population who are in transition toward a macrobiotic or more plant-centered way of eating.

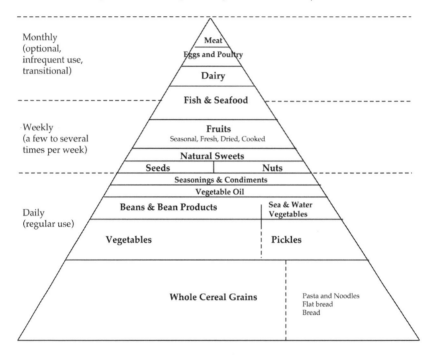

Source: *The Book of Macrobiotics: The Universal Way of Health, Happiness & Peace* by Michio Kushi. Square One Publishers.

After a mid-morning break, it was time for our cooking class in the main kitchen. We prepared our lunch in this class. The chefs who taught at the Institute were experts. Wendy Esko, one of the top macrobiotic chefs in the world, was one of our teachers. Aveline Kushi, Michio's wife, also taught cooking classes. She was amazing, having been one George Ohsawa's original students in Japan. Much later, I had the good fortune to meet George Ohsawa's wife, Lima. She was in her nineties and looked unbelievably young for her age.

We learned how to properly prepare macrobiotic foods—how to pressure-cook grains and how to chop and cut vegetables properly. Since I had been cooking for myself, I already knew how to do a lot of this, but I still learned new recipes and techniques, new ways to put things together, and new ideas that proved to be very helpful as my cooking skills improved.

Shizuko Yamamoto, author of *Shiatsu: The Whole Body Approach to Health*, came to the Institute. Shiatsu is the ancient art of acupressure massage that restores harmony between the individual and the universe. It heals by allowing the life force, Chi (qi), within all of us to flow freely. With traditional shiatsu, the person administering the massage utilizes only his or her hands and fingers. Barefoot shiatsu allows use of the feet and toes for a more balanced, deeper massage. It encourages better posture for a longer period of time, which, in turn, allows deeper breathing, enabling the shiatsu practitioner to give a better, deeper massage. Barefoot shiatsu includes not only this form of massage but also guidance on how to become healthier and more in tune with the world through proper diet, exercise, meditation, and cultivation of self-reliance. Shizuko once gave me a barefoot shiatsu massage—it was one of the most amazing experiences of my life.

I didn't meet Michio the first week I was there as he was on tour giving lectures. However, my first week was a week of learning new things and meeting some of the most dedicated and knowledgeable macrobiotic teachers in the world. I had been starving to be among like-minded people—people who understood what I was dealing with. I had come from an ordinary day-to-day world where I struggled to stay alive and had stepped into an entirely different world. Here there was absolutely no fear. I can't begin to explain what a joy that was.

During that week, I remember laughing. That may sound like a strange thing for me to recall, but I hadn't laughed in such a long time that it was an enormous release. I had been so serious, so focused on my healing, and under intense pressure. Here at the Institute, I found the companionship I craved. Here the food was so good that I felt high from eating it. All of us were laughing and having fun. Who needs to drink liquor when you feel good just from the food? And it was wonderful to be in a place where people were doing things for me. Outside of Mama's help, I had managed by myself for so long that this was a real blessing.

That week, I had a consultation with Ed Esko, the teacher who had spoken at the orientation a few days earlier. Ed had worked with Michio for many years and was very reassuring. Out of everyone at the seminar that week, I was one of the few who had been dealing with stage IV cancer. I had been through a tough time, of course, but he assured me I was doing fine. These were the very words I needed to hear, and I breathed a deep sigh of relief. One of the things he told me really got my attention. He said the most important thing anyone can do is to *be happy*. If you are not happy in your life for any reason—work, home, location, whatever—it's very important that you change either your circumstances or the way you deal with them. His words made a big impact on me. As I thought about what he said, the idea crossed my mind of possibly moving from Texas to Becket, Massachusetts, where it seemed I had found the help I needed. But I wasn't sure I had the courage to put so many miles between me and my little girl. It was one thing to go for a week-long seminar, and another to actually relocate. I dismissed the thought for the time being.

Surprisingly, no one I met at the Institute was anti-doctor or anti-medical establishment. In fact, they didn't bash anyone at all. They were all very humble and non-judgmental. And if there was ever anything I didn't understand, I could ask questions . . . and I asked plenty. I learned and absorbed everything I could while I was there. Some of my fellow students thought the macrobiotic diet itself was going to be a magic bullet. They thought they could simply eat a certain way for a few months then go back to their regular lifestyle. I knew better. I hadn't forgotten the hospital psychotherapist's warning to me: "You can't do the macrobiotic diet half way. You have to really stick with it. If you can do that, I think there's a good chance you might get well." At that time, learning about the macrobiotic diet was learning about something that 99.9-percent of people in this country knew nothing about.

The macrobiotic diet doesn't stop at your plate. It's much more than learning which foods to eat and which to avoid. It's all about yin and yang principles—learning to properly balance not just your food, but your life. The idea is to create balance, harmony, and health throughout the mind and body. We all have the same twenty-four hours a day. With eight hours devoted to sleep and eight hours devoted to work (for many of us), that leaves eight hours to take care of ourselves. And while it sometimes took me two-and-a-half hours to cook and eat a meal, it was worth it. Our food is vital in creating our healing energy, so it's not something to rush through. I learned how to cook better, tastier dishes and now had new cookbooks at my disposal. Whole grains were the staple of all meals that week with protein sources from smaller beans, like lentils, adzuki beans, and chickpeas. We also had a variety of sea vegetables and seaweed daily and tofu or tempeh a couple times that week. We didn't eat a lot of raw foods; most were cooked, but we did make pressed salads—a layering of raw vegetables, like sliced cucumbers or radishes, with a small amount of sea salt sprinkled on the top layer. The vegetables are then weighed down with a heavy plate. Essentially, you're pickling the vegetables. This process releases the water from the veggies, making them more digestible without destroying their healthful enzymes.

We ate South River brand miso soup twice a day, every day. Natural miso is traditionally prepared and has three basic characteristics: it is fermented slowly (usually six months to three years) at the natural temperature of its environment. It is made from only natural ingredients and is never pasteurized. Fermentation is the key to miso's healing properties, which are destroyed by high heat. For this reason, it's important not to overheat miso soup. Christian and Gaella Elwell, founders of South River Miso Company, had been students at the Kushi Institute. Their hand-crafted, wood-fired, organic miso was made in the centuries-old, Japanese farmhouse tradition. My body craved this food. On the macrobiotic diet, I felt like every cell in my body was dancing! For dinner Thursday night, we went to Ginga, the local macrobiotic restaurant. Because of my strict diet, I hadn't been able to eat in restaurants for quite a long time, so that night out was great fun for me.

That week at the Institute I began to realize that there was life outside Huntsville, Texas. I was among people who were sensitive to me—people who didn't think of me as a freak with cancer, which I had felt (or imagined) many of my friends back in Texas had thought of me. Here, I was treated like a real human being, not someone people were scared to get close to. The experience gave me just the lift I needed. Before I came to the Institute I had managed on my own and that independence had been good for me, but this was so much better.

I began to dare to dream a new dream. This transformative week had given me hope not only for healing, but also for going forward in life. Now I was even more positive that I would survive. And I knew that I wanted my life to count for something. It was a time of self-reflection. "I want my life to make a difference," I thought. "I don't want to sell beer and cigarettes and gasoline any more. I want to devote my life to helping others."

I wondered what it would be like to live at the Kushi Institute. When I asked Walt, the general manager, if people can enroll there for work study, he said they could if they are suited for it.

"Would it be possible for someone like me to do work study?" I asked.

"Sure!" he said. "You come on up. As long as you can do chores to help, you're fine. And you look like you can handle it. We'll give you room and board. Just give me a call when you're ready, and if you're sure it's something you really want to do." He also told me that one of the top macrobiotic writers, Alex Jack, lived in Dallas with his wife. He gave me Alex's phone number and told me to look him up.

Saturday arrived too soon, and it was time to leave. It had been a transformative week for me in many ways. After breakfast and saying our goodbyes, we were given a sack lunch of nori rolls with veggies and rice balls to tide us over on our travel home. When I got back to Dallas, I called Alex Jack, who invited me to his home for dinner. He and his wife, Gale, were very welcoming and made me feel like family. Both were teachers of macrobiotics and were experts on its philosophy and principles. Alex had authored several books on the topic. They served a delicious macrobiotic meal, just like the ones served at the Kushi Institute. "Why don't you share meals with us?" they asked. "We'd love to have you come here often. Every day if you want. This sounded great to me. I felt so lucky.

Most days after work, I would join the Jacks for dinner. I insisted upon paying for my meals, but the companionship they gave me was priceless. I now had supportive friends in Dallas who understood what living the macrobiotic lifestyle was all about.

After dinner, I would go home and practice my Dōln and visualizations. I'd go for walks or bike rides, and spend the night with my leg pump. No matter how late the hour, I did all the things I had to do for my health. Back in my running days before I got sick, I felt invincible. The lymph surgery had slowed my running down to a walk, but I still felt the need to push myself as far as I could. One day I decided to push myself with an eighteen-mile run around White Rock Lake. I told myself that if I could do that, then I'd *know* that I could get well. I wanted to prove to myself that I could do anything. So one Saturday morning, I drove out to the lake and I challenged myself to run those eighteen miles without stopping. It took everything I had to make the distance, and I was so sore afterward that I could barely walk for nearly two weeks. But I did it! And meeting that challenge strengthened my resolve even more as I went forward.

One evening at dinner, I learned that the general manager at the Institute had resigned and Alex had been offered the position. He and Gale were moving to Becket. Alex knew that I had been interested in the work study program there and suggested that I join them on staff. I knew the move would mean a lot of changes in my life. What about my little girl? I knew there was no possibility of Mellisa and I getting back together, but was I going to be able to see Carol as much as I wanted (and needed) if I moved to the East Coast? I had loved being at the Institute and even entertained the idea of moving there, but it's a different thing to actually be faced with the decision. I decided to go off by myself to think things over. I drove to Santa Fe, New Mexico, and found a motel with a kitchenette where I could cook for myself and spend a long weekend considering my situation. Santa Fe was one of my favorite places. I felt it was where I could search deep within myself to discover my path.

For three days I debated the pros and cons of moving to the East Coast and enrolling in the Institute's work-study program. I knew that if I was going to have any chance of being around for my daughter for the long-term, I had to do all I could to regain my health. I would visit my little girl as often as possible and be there for her as best I could. It might be a long journey, but the faster I got well, the better it would be. My logic said I needed to go. My heart, not so much. Still, if I was going to remain on this earth for her, I felt I needed to pursue every opportunity to get better, wherever that took me. When I informed my business associates in Houston of my decision they understood that I needed to put my health first. I was enormously grateful for their support.

Saying good-bye to my daughter was one of the hardest things I've ever done. I could not control my tears. But leaving her made me more determined to do everything within my power to recover my health as fast as possible. I wanted to see her grow up and, more importantly, not leave her fatherless at an early age. Mellisa was overseeing the businesses we had built, which enabled her to provide for our little girl. So I got rid of all my personal possessions except my trusty Jeep and a couple of suitcases. It was time to move forward.

I knew instinctively that it was going to be a very exciting journey filled with new challenges. One of my suitcases contained supplies: a hot plate, non-perishable macrobiotic food, dried seaweed, brown rice, and other grains. As I drove cross country from Texas to Massachusetts, I cooked my food in motel rooms. When possible, I would stop at local health food stores and pick up the fresh greens and vegetables I needed for that night's meal.

Each evening, by the time I got to my motel room, I would be ravenous. I'd cover the smoke alarm–just in case—as I cooked my simple one-dish meal. I always made enough so that I'd have leftovers the next day for lunch, which I usually ate by the side of the road. Then I would lie on the floor and do my Dōln stretches. Each morning, I would walk at least forty-five minutes as I practiced deep breathing. I'd take a deep breath, hold it for three to four seconds, then release. I'd do this for at least ten minutes during my walks and it always made me feel better. I did my best to stick with my routine even though I was traveling. I was determined not to cut any corners. I definitely wasn't going to take time off from taking care of myself just because I was on the road.

Five days later, on a cold and snowy February day, I arrived in Becket. The drive through the Berkshires was every bit as beautiful during the winter as it had been in the fall. The lakes and ponds were frozen over and I could see ice fisherman enjoying their sport. The area surrounding the Institute was even more picturesque than I remembered. Both Aveline Kushi and Alex Jack greeted me and instantly I felt right at home.

My work-study position involved various chores at the Institute. Cutting firewood in the forest and bringing it to the main house was one of my outdoor jobs. Fortunately, I had managed to regain my strength since leaving the hospital. I was a little on the thin side, but so much better—and for sure, I knew my way around a chainsaw. And as long as I stayed active, my leg continued to improve every day. I also washed dishes twice a day. Many days, there were up to forty people in the house sharing meals. I had never washed so many dishes in my life! But I was so grateful to be there, I would have done anything.

The Kushi Institute sat on six-hundred acres. Because I liked to walk so much, soon I knew all the trails and back roads in the area like I knew the back of my hand. I enjoyed being out in nature. I found it very healing to walk barefoot on the earth and even in the morning snow on occasion (that would sure get me going!). The Appalachian Trail was nearby, and I loved to hike it. Sometimes when I'd come across a creek or stream in the mountains, I would lie down next to it—even in the snow—and feel the warm sunshine on my face. To me, it was paradise. I'd walk several miles a day like clockwork, whether there was snow, rain, sleet, or black ice on the ground. I can't remember a day when I missed it, and I always did my deep breathing when I walked. I learned that oxygen kills cancer cells . . . so I knew how important these daily walks were.

I had read about Native Americans sleeping directly on the ground and how healing it was, so I decided to give it a try. I had a small tent that I'd often pitch behind the main house and sleep in, even in the wintertime. I felt so much better sleeping on the earth. But after a while, I was asked to stop. I guess it may have looked a little odd for a staff member to be sleeping outside in a tent.

At one time, the dormitory where I and most of the staff normally slept had been a monastery. The rooms were very small with just enough room for a futon and a small clothes closet. There was also one window to crack open to get some fresh air and a peek at the New England landscape. I remember lying in my room and thinking I could almost hear the chants of the monks from years past. Speaking of chants, I learned different ones at the Institute to energize the body's chakras. One of the staff members taught Kundalini yoga classes that I participated in at 5:30 before breakfast. Kundalini yoga is like an express train that shakes and wakes you up. It's an ancient art in which Kundalini energy is awakened and summoned up the spine through energy centers of the body. I remember, in particular, practicing the often exhausting Breath of Fire exercise, which is done with this type of yoga. With it, breathing, which is rapid, rhythmic, and continuous, is done through the nostrils with the mouth closed. There is an equal amount of breath on the inhale and exhale, with no pause in between. Very heating and detoxifying, the Breath of Fire energizes the whole body.

As before, I continued to chew my food 180 times per mouthful. I guess you could say this became my meditation. In fact, there were times when I wanted to eat alone instead of with a group so that I could meditate in complete peace and quiet while chewing. I would sit on the old chair in my room with my legs crossed in a meditative position and chew my food with my eyes closed. This opened me up to another level of meditation. I was now focused on consciously being in total control of my own destiny. I was also determined to set a good example, both for myself and for others.

While I was at the Institute, I saw many people whose health was transformed, as my own had been. I recalled the long days and nights spent in the hospital, my first attempts to learn how to cook my own macrobiotic food, and the healing I had experienced along the way. I'll never forget waking up one morning back in Dallas after about three months of following the macrobiotic diet and discovering the bed sheets were wet. When I lifted the covers, I saw a dark, graphite-colored liquid oozing out of both of my legs, midway between my knees and my ankles. To me it was as if the cancer, the poison in my body, was finding a way out all on its own. It seeped from a pinhole size opening on both of my legs for quite a while, then just simply stopped, never to happen again. I had come a long way. Life can be a battle. Cancer is a bigger battle.

One day, Alex told me they needed a new operations manager. He said, "I know you have a business background and I'd like to offer the position to you. You've been great to have around and have done a great job for us. If you want this position, we could pay you a small salary in addition to your room and board." It wasn't a lot of money, but it was enough to buy gas and maybe go to the movies on weekends. I took the job.

As operations manager, my job included purchasing all the food and supplies for the Institute. I would drive out to the local organic farms and make deals with the farmers for produce. It was an adventure and I felt like I was helping people by finding the very best food possible. In the wintertime when there was no fresh harvest on the farms, I'd shop at the large health food store, which was about an hour's drive away, to buy organic foods in bulk. I was also in charge of purchasing the heating fuel for the buildings, and I made sure there was plenty of firewood available. I was busy, working all the time, and I loved it.

The residential seminars were ongoing and I made arrangements for the guests who were traveling back and forth to the Institute and needed transportation. Sometimes I would assign a driver to make runs to the airport or bus station, but I enjoyed picking up many of the guests myself, using the company pickup truck. As neither Michio nor his wife drove, I would often drive them wherever they needed to go. Michio continued to travel around the world, giving lectures everywhere he went. When he was at the Institute, he would see clients all day long. He would examine them in his traditional way of looking at their faces, eyes, hands, and feet and make recommendations as to diet and lifestyle adjustments for whatever their condition happened to be.

Driving staff and guests, lecturers and students back and forth gave me the opportunity to get to know them even better. I met a lot of interesting people including Dr. Anthony Sattilaro, whose book *Recalled by Life* had influenced me so much. I consider it one of the books that saved my life. I met a number of other well-known healers such as Dr. Patch Adams, Shizuko Yamamoto, and Herman Aihara, a well-respected pioneer in the macrobiotic movement. But it was the people who were sick and came to the Institute as a last resort that I related to the most. These were people from all walks of life who were experiencing the same fears that I had. I could see it on their faces when I picked them up at the airport or bus station for the first day of their residential seminar. Many had been through the mill, were at the end of their rope, and didn't know where else to turn. I would sometimes share my story and the important things I had learned. It always made feel good to be able to inspire others. It always gave me great pleasure to see their improvement at the end of their week-long stay.

Most of our visitors left with a new-found hope. They were excited and felt they had a chance of surviving whatever it was they were dealing with. It made me feel like all of us at the Institute were instrumental in changing lives, and I felt like I was where I was supposed to be. As luck would have it, I met a man named Herb Shapiro at the Institute. Years later, it was Herb who led me to yet another healing experience, but I'll get to that a little later.

One thing I've noticed is that many of the people I've met who have cancer are the nicest people you could ever meet. Do we hold our emotions in? Did we not handle stress well? I was learning that being in a constant state of stress or fear is very harmful to the body. Major stress suppresses the immune system. Traumatic events from the past can cause some people to feel trapped and unable to escape from the painful memory of the experience. Levels of cortisol, the stress hormone, remain high, directly suppressing the immune system. When the immune system isn't operating at peak performance, cancer cells are left to grow exponentially.

Sometimes I wondered why the macrobiotic diet worked so well for me, but not for everyone who came to the Institute. Cancer is very complex and each person is different. People were at different stages of their illness when they arrived. Maybe for some, it was simply too little too late. I remember Michio saying that he could only give those who are sick the building blocks of health, and that it was up to them to take it from there. He was right. We cannot expect anyone else to make us healthy. I had come so close to dying that I didn't dare take anything for granted. I worked very hard at healing. In addition, I wanted to be alert to any new avenues of healing. After all, the macrobiotic lifestyle had once been a brand new idea for me!

One day, I was talking to a friend of mine at the Institute about doing something more for my health. Although I was feeling pretty good at that time, I wondered if there was something I should be adding to my regimen. If there was, I wasn't sure what it could be. I wanted to be open to anything and everything to continue improving my health. My friend was a brilliant man, a renowned macrobiotic teacher who had graduated from Harvard. He told me about the Rudolph Steiner philosophy.

Rudolph Steiner was a German philosopher and founder of the biodynamic approach to agriculture—the first intentional form of organic farming. He was a highly trained scientist and respected philosopher. Later in his life, he came to prominence for his spiritual-scientific approach to knowledge called *anthroposophy*. The guiding principle of anthroposophic healthcare is recognizing the autonomy and dignity of patients and helping them help themselves. Self-responsibility is addressed, and therapeutic goals are to stimulate different forms of self-healing. The aim is to strengthen the whole constitution of the sick patient by taking into account all dimensions: physical, emotional, mental, spiritual, and social.

"You know, James, I agree with you," my friend said. "Maybe you should look at other healing modalities, too. There's such a thing as being too strict for too long and not getting enough fat and protein in your diet. A cancer diet needs to be strict to help detoxify and take a load off the immune system so that you can then rebuild, but it may not be the right diet for rebuilding." That got my attention. My friend recommended a local anthroposophical doctor—an M.D. who was Rudolph Steiner-trained. The doctor believed in a healthy lifestyle and bringing an unhealthy body back into balance. He recommended Iscador, an extract of mistletoe, to rebuild my immune system. The extract had been a popular natural remedy in treating cancer in Europe for years. I was willing to try it. I had learned so much, come so far, and nothing sounded outrageous to me now. The Iscador was to be injected in the area around (not directly in) my spleen. After the doctor showed me how to do the injections I thought, "Oh boy. How much fun is this going to be, sticking myself with needles every day?" But I did it. I ordered the Iscador from Germany, which was sent to me as samples, and injected it as the doctor had shown me twice a day for an entire year. "After that," the doctor said, "You probably won't need to do it anymore."

When I first started the injections, and as the Iscador began to work, I knew my immune system had kicked in when I started feeling flu-like symptoms. After a month or so, the uncomfortable symptoms went away. As recommended, I continued the treatments for an entire year and felt stronger and stronger as time went on. No one else at the Institute knew what I was doing. I felt like a renegade but kept it to myself. It was a bold thing to do, but I was determined to do all I could to help myself.

I lived and worked at the Kushi Institute for nearly four years. While it had been a wonderful experience and was very healing for me, the feeling that there was something else I needed to do for my health, for myself, became even stronger. Was I going to live at the Institute forever? Was I going to sleep in this little room with only a futon and a chair forever? Was I ever going to have a business again? What was my life going to look like in the next twenty years? These are some of the questions that went through my mind.

Learning about and living the macrobiotic lifestyle had been one of the greatest experiences of my life. It transformed me into a more enlightened, healthy individual. It not only changed my life, it saved my life. I have enormous gratitude for Michio, Aveline, Alex Jack, Ed Esko, and all the teachers and staff members that I became close to at the Institute. They had welcomed me with open arms. If it hadn't been for them, I probably wouldn't be around today. But my heart was telling me it was time to move on.

During my time at the Institute, I had kept in touch with Carol, my little girl, through frequent phone calls, cards, letters, and visits to Texas as often as I could. Every year on her birthday, I'd send her the prettiest dress I could find. I think she still has a few of those dresses. A couple years into my stay at the Institute, Mellisa and I finalized our divorce. I had signed over the businesses to her, which provided for her and our daughter. I didn't have a lot of money, but I still had a small ski house that we had purchased in Breckenridge, Colorado, and that Mellisa had agreed I would keep. I decided it would be my next destination. I planned to fix up the house and then sell it. Besides, the chance to live in the Rocky Mountains was something I had always looked forward to.

So with a fond farewell and a huge debt of gratitude to everyone at the Kushi Institute, I loaded up my trusty Jeep with my few belongings and headed to Texas to visit my little girl before making the trip to Colorado. God, how I missed her! Mellisa was doing a good job caring for our daughter, and I knew she was in good hands. Phone calls, cards, and letters had their place, but that face-to-face time was precious. Deep within my spirit, I felt that I was doing what I needed to do not only for myself, but for Carol. The years have a way of working things out. Little did I know at that time there was much in store for my daughter and me—working as a team—down the road.

I would criss-cross the country a couple times before taking the next big leap in my healing journey and come face-to-face with the love of my life—and the most amazing health warrior I had ever known.

6

Guess What
Came to Dinner?

"How sweet it is to love someone, how right it is to care.
How long it's been since yesterday, and what about tomorrow . . ."
—JOHN DENVER, FROM *POEMS, PRAYERS, AND PROMISES*

Arriving in Breckenridge, Colorado, I was even more excited about the possibilities ahead. I finally felt like I didn't have one foot in the grave as had been predicted when I first was diagnosed with cancer. I was able to relax a little and start to dream again. When you come face to face with death as I did, the last thing you're worried about is planning for your financial future. You're just struggling to stay alive. At last, I felt as though I might actually be able to be there for my daughter for the long term. My journey into the macrobiotic way of life had benefited me in many ways, not the least of which was the way it had helped me to become even more disciplined with my diet and exercise routine. It had saved my life. I was grateful to be stronger now, but I was still very strict on the macrobiotic program. I was determined not to cut corners or to settle back into my old eating patterns.

Living and working at the Kushi Institute had been a wonderful experience at the time in my life when I needed it most. I now better understood the changes in diet and lifestyle that were required to regain control of my health. I also learned a great deal from the people who came to the Institute in search of answers for their own health issues. When it comes to our individual healthcare, too many of us are willing to hand over the responsibility to others without hesitation—until we discover the system we have trusted really doesn't have an answer. Each and every guest at the Institute, including me, came to the realization that the responsibility for our well-being begins with ourselves.

As time went on, I continued to grow in strength. When the cancer didn't rear its ugly head as before, I began to give myself permission to think about the possibilities ahead. Back in the land of the living, I took a good hard look at where I was in life. I knew that it took money to be independent. I also knew I was running out of money and needed to figure out a course of action. I had willingly signed over most of what I owned to Mellisa in the divorce, but I still had our ski house in Breckenridge, along with the Texas property I had inherited. I decided that it was time to sell the Colorado house to generate a little income.

Breckenridge had been a favorite vacation spot for several years. I've always been particularly fond of skiing and loved it there. I looked forward to spending a little time there while getting the ski house ready to sell. There were some repairs that needed to be made before putting it on the market, so I got busy. In addition, I looked for any part-time work I could find. There weren't many high-paying jobs in the area at that time nor were there many low-paying jobs, but that didn't stop me. I applied for anything and everything I could find, but with no luck. I even remember applying for a job delivering flowers for five dollars an hour. The owner of the florist shop said he thought I was overqualified and probably wouldn't stick around very long, and he turned me down.

With no job, I was able to focus entirely on making the minor repairs that were needed and taking care of my health. I went ahead and listed the property with a local realtor even though I hadn't made all of the needed repairs. I figured it might take some time to sell. Once again, I was back to doing my own cooking and fending for myself. In the mornings, I would fix a macrobiotic breakfast with whole grains, miso soup, and vegetables. I loved to spend time outdoors. Often, I would pack up leftovers from the night before and spend the whole day hiking in the high mountains, often up to twenty miles a day. The Rocky Mountains are incredibly beautiful and very rugged. I was addicted to being out in nature. It was summertime in Colorado, which meant it was chilly in the mornings and very comfortable in the afternoons. My kind of weather! I also loved to drive and explore the area. Sometimes I would stop and pitch my tent for the night and cook outdoors. I still had my trusty Coleman camp stove that had served me well in Texas a few years back.

While I was loving every minute of my time in Colorado, I missed the companionship of like-minded people. I made friends with the guy at the health food store in town as I was there nearly every day, but that was about the only friend I had made there. I spent a lot of my time thinking, meditating, and wondering what to do next. Don't get me wrong, it may have been a lonely life, but it was a very valuable experience. I wouldn't trade it for anything. I came to realize that life is not meant to be so full of stress and a burden to endure. From watching the wild animals roaming the mountainside, I realized they tended to their own needs—they ate and drank what they needed to simply sustain life. Why do we humans load ourselves down with so much stress? Is it really necessary? I felt particularly close to God and nature during my time there.

One day in the middle of September, I decided to make what I call a "vision quest" where I could be alone in nature and where I could try to get a handle on my direction in life, what I needed to do next in my healing journey. I decided the best place for me to do that was in the high mountains. So I packed up my Jeep with my pup tent and backpack and headed for one of my favorite places high in the Rockies outside Telluride. A former silver mining camp on the San Miguel River, Telluride sits in a box canyon surrounded by steep forested mountains and cliffs. I drove as high as I could, then parked my Jeep at a campground before hiking even further up the mountain. I was almost 14,000 feet above sea level and it was *really* cold at night, often dropping into the teens. Sometimes I would wake up to a dusting of snow on my pup tent. I would often encounter thunderstorms at night with lightning that was so close I thought it would surely hit me. I could hear the rain pelting down as I slept. It's a whole different world when you're experiencing nature on such close terms.

I encountered all types of wildlife while hiking, but rarely encountered another person. I saw deer, elk, and an occasional bear. Sometimes I would sit or lie down near a stream or river during the warm afternoon or early evening. All kinds of animals would come to the stream to drink and not feel threatened, even though I was very near. Occasionally I would hear and see a plane or jet fly overhead. I was so high up the mountain, I felt like I could almost reach out and grab them.

The week of my vision quest was a very special time for me. I was full of gratitude—for my little girl, for my improved health, and for this opportunity to spend time in one of my favorite places on the planet. I can still see myself cooking over an open fire, fighting the wind and the elements, and looking forward to sleeping in my small tent. I felt so close to God up in those high mountains. There is nothing better than sitting on a rock and viewing the sunset over the top of 14,000-foot-high snow-capped mountains. If that's not close to God, nothing is. During that week, I did a lot of soul searching, hoping to find direction in my life. I had an unmistakable, very strong urge to go back to New England. For reasons I didn't fully understand at the time, I felt that if I went back to the East Coast, I would find the answers that would carry me forward in life. I felt as if I had some unfinished business there, though I didn't know what it was. But after that unforgettable week in the high mountains, I felt unimaginably calm and had a better handle on my new direction. I packed up my tent and went back to my Breckenridge home.

Isn't it funny how things come together once you've learned to trust your intuition and have found your purpose in life? When I got back to my ski house, I first called my little girl. It was great to hear her voice; she seemed to be doing well. I then checked the answering machine for any messages I had missed during the past week. One message was from the realtor I had listed my house with. "I've been trying to get hold of you," he said. "I have someone who is very interested in your property. Please call me as soon as possible." I called the next morning. Even though I wasn't quite finished with the minor repairs and all the little things that needed to be done on the house, the realtor wanted to show it to the prospective buyer. The buyer wanted to purchase a home for her son, who was setting up a business in town. On the prospective buyer's first walk-through of the house, she said, "I love it. This is perfect!" In fact, she didn't even care about the little repairs I hadn't yet made. The sale went through faster than I had anticipated and the buyer wanted me out within thirty days. My financial troubles were over for the time being and thanks to the introspective week I had spent in the mountains, I knew where I was supposed to go.

I placed a call to my good friend Paula Breen, a congregational minister I had met while working at the Kushi Institute. She lived in the Berkshires and often went to the Institute as a guest to share meals and take an occasional class. I told her I was headed back her way. Without hesitation she offered to let me hang my hat at her place. So I packed my few belongings, got in my Jeep, and drove back across the country. When I got to Paula's, I discovered she had another houseguest. It was her boyfriend, who just happened to also be my friend, Herb Shapiro. Herb lived in New Jersey and was there visiting Paula. Paula was a gracious host. My contribution to the living arrangement was cooking for all of us, and I enjoyed it immensely. By that time, I had become a pretty good macrobiotic cook. At times I even entertained the idea of cooking for a living.

Herb and his brother, Steve, owned a successful chain of health food stores in Morristown, Chester, Parsippany, and Montclair, New Jersey. Whenever one brother was away, whether for business or for pleasure, the other brother managed the stores. Knowing I needed a job, Herb invited me to work at one of his stores. I thought it was a great idea. Not only would it allow me to learn about the health food business (I knew Herb could teach me a lot), it would also be more in tune with my consciousness and new way of life.

So after a few days at Paula's place, Herb and I headed to his apartment in Mt. Arlington, New Jersey. Herb was always willing to talk and to listen and was a very good friend to me. Of anyone I've ever met, he was the most knowledgeable about the health food business. As we traveled, we talked and got to know each other even better. I learned about his relationship with Paula, which had gotten stronger over time. He tried to visit her as much as possible. When he asked about my relationship with women, I told him about my divorce and that I wasn't really seeing anyone. I was too wrapped up in my healing journey for much else.

I asked Herb why he got into health food stores since he seemed to be so involved with the macrobiotic lifestyle. He felt that there was more than one answer to maintaining good health. "Besides," he said. "It's a good way to make a living, as long as you hire the right people." I knew that was true, based on my own experience in running my own stores in the past. He also told me that he spent a great deal of his time meeting and greeting customers and answering their questions. I told Herb I was excited about the prospect of working with him. I really valued the opportunity and looked forward to learning whatever he could teach me about the health food industry. It was going to be an exciting adventure. I looked forward to being involved in a new career, to learning about a new business, and to spending time with my friend.

During the course of our conversation, Herb mentioned a really good nutritionist he was seeing. Her name was Ann Louise Gittleman and he had originally learned about her from her books, which she carried in his stores. "She's amazing," Herb said. "I've never met anyone as knowledgeable as she is when it comes to anything related to nutrition and health. I'll introduce her to you sometime. It sounded good to me! I looked forward to meeting her. After all, anyone who knew as much about health as she did was someone I'd like to get to know!

After arriving at Herb's place, it only took a few days to get into a routine. I would get up each morning and cook breakfast for the two of us before going to work at the store. Since I had owned and managed my own stores in the past, this was a good fit for me. I helped stock products, kept the store clean, and worked behind the counter as needed. At night, I would come home and cook a big macrobiotic dinner, with plenty of left-overs for lunch the next day. I did that for about nine months. I loved the experience and Herb treated me like family. What more could I ask? We lived in a small town with plenty of hills. I walked every day and continued to do the deep breathing on my walks. On weekends, I'd go hiking. I became close friends with a woman who was a member of the Appalachian Mountain Club and we often hiked together, sometimes fifteen to eighteen miles a day. It was the next best thing to being in the Rockies.

As time went on, however, I began to notice that I didn't feel as well in New Jersey as I had felt at the Institute. I wondered if I was getting sick again. Why was I so achy all over? I would sometimes feel as though I had the flu. I hadn't felt that way since those experimental cancer treatments back in Texas. I noticed that when I went away on weekends or hiked in the Catskill Mountains, I would feel better. But when I'd come back to the house in New Jersey, within a couple of days, I'd feel lousy again. Herb confided that he hadn't been feeling that great either. Then I figured it out. In addition to living near a nuclear facility, we lived two miles as the crow flies from Picatinny Arsenal, a military research and manufacturing facility. A couple miles in the other direction, there was a gun powder plant. In other words, we were living right in the middle of a polluted, toxic area. I knew I needed to leave for the sake of my health.

So when Herb decided to go to Stockbridge, Massachusetts, to spend the winter with Paula in a house he had rented there, and asked if I'd like to come along, I found his offer very inviting. "It's a big, beautiful place," he said, "and there's plenty of room. We can stay there for the entire winter season, except for a couple weeks at Christmas when the owner wants to stay there. Why don't you join us and, of course, you can do the cooking." He said that I could either stay in New Jersey and work at his store, or I could come to Stockbridge and he would pay me to cook for them. It didn't take long for me to decide that spending the winter with my friends in Stockbridge was what I wanted to do.

One day that winter, Herb asked, "Do you remember the nutritionist I told you about? Ann Louise Gittleman? Well, as it turns out, she is holding a seminar next weekend at a hotel in the Berkshires. Why don't you come along, and I'll pay your way?" I looked forward to going.

The seminar was on the subject of intestinal parasites. Ann Louise was a very good speaker and held everyone's attention. I was intrigued. She talked about parasites and their connection to health and disease, mentioning that they can often be one of the causes of cancer and immune problems. That really got my attention. After the lecture, Herb introduced me to her. I told her how much I enjoyed her talk, and then mentioned that I'd had cancer. Then I said, "You know, after hearing you speak, I'm wondering if I have parasites. Do you think I might?"

She paused, studied my face, and said, "Yes, I think you do."

Wow, I thought. "How do you know?" I asked.

"Well, you have that parasitic look," was her answer. Instantly I recalled the times I would take my dogs to the vet and the first thing the vet would do was to check for worms, which they'd usually test positive for. I remember de-worming my cattle on an annual basis. After hearing Ann Louise's lecture, I learned that parasites are known for greatly suppressing the body's immune system. Much later, she explained to me that the grayish-tinge around my mouth was a dead giveaway for a parasitic infection.

"Look," she said. "Don't take my word for it. You should go get checked out. There is a world-renowned Columbian parasitologist, Dr. Herman Bueno, practicing in New York City. I haven't met him," she said, "but I'd like to. I would be happy to ride along with you if you want to go see him." Wow, I thought. Here is Ann Louise Gittleman, a brilliant woman, writer, speaker, expert in cutting-edge natural health, and she's willing to go *with me* to meet one of the best parasitologists in the world. Then I immediately thought, "Oh God, here is this beautiful woman telling me I look to her like I have parasites." I put aside my male ego and said, "Yes! I'll take you up on that."

At one of Herb's appointments with Ann Louise, he learned that she was looking for a new place to live. She had been sharing a house with a friend in the Berkshires, but her roommate was soon to be moving out West, leaving Ann Louise with an unmanageable expense and the need to move quickly. Herb invited her to stay as one of his guests at the Stockbridge house, and she traded nutrition consulting in exchange for room and board. There was plenty of room in the house, which had once been a bed and breakfast inn. The day Ann Louise got there, I helped her move in. As fate would have it, her room was across from mine.

Remembering Ann Louise's suggestion that I be tested for parasites, I made an appointment with Dr. Bueno. The date of my appointment soon rolled around and Ann Louise and I drove to New York City. As soon as I met Dr. Bueno, I was immediately put at ease by his great bedside manner. I told him I'd had cancer, how I'd met Ann Louise, and that I wanted to get checked out for parasites.

"No problem," he said. "Let's get a sample and see how you're doing." He took a rectal tissue swab sample, made slides, and used a teaching microscope so we could simultaneously see what he was looking at. The whole process didn't take long at all.

"Ok, my friend," he said in a soothing tone of voice. "Let's go over what I'm finding here. You're loaded with *entamoeba histolytica*, a one-celled organism, the kind of thing you pick up in Mexico and many other foreign countries. It can really make you sick. You also have *giardia lamblia*, another one-celled organism, which is a parasite you can get from drinking water from lakes and streams, often in mountainous areas. It can really cause havoc. You also have *ascaris lumbricoides*, round worms. Round worms? That rang a bell. Many of my animals back in Texas had suffered with them.

Dr. Bueno continued, "I'm not surprised at these results. *I have never seen a case of cancer or AIDS in my whole career that didn't have a parasitic involvement.*" He felt it was one of the major underlying causes of disease that too often was overlooked.

To rid myself of the parasites, Dr. Bueno recommended a certain herbal formula he had developed. He said that drugs aren't as effective in the long term and that herbs work much better than anything else he had found. "But you'll have to stay on the regimen for a while, maybe three months or even more to get rid of all that you have in your system." He recommended I come back in three months to get checked out again. On the drive home, I thought a lot about everything the doctor had said. If parasites were an underlying cause of cancer as he seemed to think, what about all the people I'd met at the Kushi Institute and at the hospital where I'd been treated? If Dr. Bueno was right, parasites could be one of the biggest problems affecting our health! It hit me like nothing had hit me in a long time.

I began the herbal formula as directed, but I just didn't feel good and it gave me really bad headaches—like someone was hitting me in the head every two seconds with a ball peen hammer. When I mentioned this to Ann Louise, I discovered that she had helped develop other herbal formulas to remedy infections. When I switched to her recommended formula, the headaches went away immediately. In addition to taking this new herbal remedy, I drank mugwort tea two to three times a day and ate a lot of raw pumpkin seeds daily after learning that both are helpful in killing intestinal worms.

I detoxed like crazy. I could hardly believe what my body was eliminating. It certainly wasn't pleasant, but it was proof that the combination of remedies was working. No doubt about it; what was coming out of my body looked just like what I had seen after my animals had been de-wormed all those years ago. But how did I contract all those parasites? I recalled those times I had been to Mexico for vacations or would drive across the Texas-Mexico border just to eat out. Then there were all those raw salads I had eaten during my running days. And I had taken care of my cows, hogs, dogs, and cats on the farm in Texas for years. I hadn't been careful to drink filtered water. Yes, there were plenty of ways I could have contracted those parasites.

After three months on the herbal program, I went back to Dr. Bueno for a checkup and was thrilled when he found no evidence of parasites. I felt much better, my digestion had improved, and I had even started to gain weight again. My health was improving, and I no longer looked like a starving refugee. I felt like my life was at last starting to make sense. Now I understood why I had been drawn back to the East Coast. Not only did I learn about one of the underlying causes of cancer and other chronic diseases during my journey here, I also met Ann Louise.

I found Ann Louise to be a very interesting person and she had a lot of friends who would often drop by to visit. She and I would often walk together in the mornings. I enjoyed our conversations and just being in her company. There was never a dull moment when she was around. When I spoke to Herb about her, he told me she was seeing someone at the time. "Well," I thought "at least we can be friends . . . for now."

One day, a guy named Len, a professional writer and friend of Ann Louise, dropped by to visit. We were all sitting around talking, and I was telling him a little about my health journey and how a book review article from a magazine had been the catalyst for the journey that saved my life. Len asked, "What book was it?"

"*The Kamikaze Cowboy* by Dirk Benedict," I told him.

"Seriously?" Len said. "I wrote that book review for the magazine!"

You could have knocked me over with a feather. Here was the guy who had opened the door to my new way of living. Talk about a small world!

At Christmastime, we had to vacate the house for two weeks as per Herb's previous agreement with the owner. Herb and Paula were going to New Jersey for those two weeks, and Paula told me and Ann Louise that we were more than welcome to stay at her permanent residence (a few towns away) while she was gone. So the two of us moved into Paula's house during the interim. Those were two very magical weeks for me. Ann Louise and I had become good friends, but now that we were all alone, we became even closer. One thing soon led to another, and our friendship blossomed into a romance. I was thrilled to be with this wonderful woman, a true health warrior, who was teaching me so much and was so very influential in my health journey. She practiced what she preached and worked tirelessly to help educate others. On the surface, we were total opposites. I'm a Texan and she's an East Coast girl. I'm an outdoor guy and she is all about nutrition, research, teaching others, and avoiding overnight stays in tents. But we found that sharing the same core beliefs bound us together.

My healing journey had taken a decidedly new turn. The information I had gathered, and the experiences I had been through, had taken me to a new level of understanding. I felt like my time on the East Coast had come to an end, and that now was the time I was supposed to go back to Santa Fe—a city that had always held a special place in my heart. I had often gone there in the past and found inner peace through my deep conversations with a Higher Power. I wasn't sure if Ann Louise was willing to go with me, but to my intense relief and pleasure, she said yes. In fact, she wanted to introduce me to the person who had been most instrumental in her decision to be a nutritionist, Dr. Hazel Parcells, who lived in Albuquerque.

After saying good-bye to our friends, we packed up our things—me in my Jeep and Ann Louise in her car—and she followed me to Santa Fe. We rented a small, but beautiful adobe house where we set up a small office space. I'll never forget the night I woke up with the idea of *Uni Key Health*. It had come to me in a dream and filled me with excitement. "Uni Key" stood for the "universal key" to health, and Uni Key Health would involve uncovering and correcting the root cause of the body's health issues.

When I began this new business, I decided to start by helping people address one of the biggest contributing factors of immunosuppression—parasites. Little did I know at that time, how big the business would eventually become. Ann Louise continued her work as a nutritionist in Santa Fe and saw clients in our home office. She would test clients for parasites and we'd send the samples to a lab. If they tested positive, I'd help the clients get rid of the parasites by recommending the appropriate herbal formulas, just as Dr. Bueno had done for me. Uni Key Health came to life! Word soon got out, and before we knew it, Ann Louise and I were very busy.

I was getting stronger and stronger and could feel the difference that getting rid of those parasites had made in my body. I had regained much of my strength and was able to run again. Although I still had the leg pump, I had gotten so healthy I didn't need it much more. I loved to go for daily runs on the beautiful Santa Fe mornings. I began to notice, however, that when I'd get back home, I'd feel a tightness in my upper shoulders and upper back and feel achy throughout my body. It almost felt like I had a slight case of the flu. What's going on? I knew there was radiation in the air and water in Los Alamos, which (as the crow flies) was not much more than twenty miles or so away from where we lived. And from my experience in New Jersey, I wondered if that was causing the achiness I was feeling. Could the radiation from Los Alamos affect us in Santa Fe? These were the questions going through my mind . . . and I was learning to pay attention to my intuition.

There is a bigger place for me in life, I thought once again. I had always wanted to set an example and minister to others. I sure didn't want anyone else to unnecessarily go through the hell I had gone through.

With Ann Louise by my side, I knew I was on the right path at last. The next leg of my health journey would lead me to Dr. Hazel Parcells, who had been one of Ann Louise's most influential teachers many years before. Dr. Parcells was a feisty woman who was over a hundred years young when I had the privilege of meeting her. She had a twinkle in her eye and a lot to teach me. Her recommendation for a radical change in my diet thrust me into an entirely new way of thinking. Her candor and down-to-earth, commonsense approach to life was exactly what I needed. My journey to fully recover my health was about to take yet another fascinating turn for the better. I was ready for it and could not have been more excited.

7

Meeting the
Teacher's Teacher

"Most of the important things in the world have been
accomplished by people who have kept on trying
when there seemed to be no hope at all."
—DALE CARNEGIE

Dr. Hazel Parcells had been one of Ann Louise's most influential mentors. When Ann Louise was twenty-five years old, she was introduced to Dr. Parcells through a health-conscious friend who showed her an ad for an upcoming seminar at the Parcells School of Scientific Nutrition in Albuquerque, New Mexico. The ad said, "If this week doesn't change your life forever, we will refund your money." That was no marketing gimmick, it was the truth. The class had indeed changed the direction of Ann Louise's life, pointing her in the direction of where and how to search for underlying causes of disease, at a time when few others were doing this. Dr. Parcells also encouraged Ann Louise to go back to school and get a degree in nutrition, which she did and which started her on the path she has been on all these years since. Meeting and getting to know Dr. Parcells would soon change my life, as well.

Ann Louise talked about Dr. Parcells frequently and always wanted to introduce me to her. So we drove to Albuquerque to spend some time with "The Doctor" as the legendary teacher and healer was familiarly known. I wasn't sure what to expect as Dr. Parcells was over 100 years old when I met her. The mental picture I had was of a fragile little old lady sitting in a rocking chair or maybe even a wheelchair. Boy, was I wrong!

Dr. Parcells greeted us upon our arrival. Her red hair and rosy cheeks were evidence of her Irish heritage. Vibrant and witty, she had the enthusiasm and energy of someone half her age . . . and she certainly wasn't wasting the time away in a rocking chair. Born in 1889, Dr. Parcells grew up on a ranch just outside Glenwood Springs, Colorado. She loved to tell stories about her life and I loved listening to her.

She said she found her calling in life after hearing the words: "Sorry, but there is nothing more we can do" from the medical experts at that time. It was the 1920s and Dr. Parcells was about forty years old. She was working in her beauty salon and could no longer ignore the fact that she was not feeling well. Each day brought on a new symptom, but she had no idea why. When the pain became nearly unbearable, she knew she had to get medical attention. Her husband had been an officer in World War I, so she was eligible to be treated at a military hospital. She went to the Fitzsimmons Army Hospital in Denver, where she was diagnosed with tuberculosis. Her condition was more serious than she even dreamed. X-rays confirmed that her right kidney was two-thirds gone, her lungs were hemorrhaging, her heart was enlarged, and one of the heart valves was damaged. The doctor told her that there was "nothing they could do" and advised her to get her things in order because her condition would not improve. He suggested she stay in a government sanitarium for the terminally ill where she would be kept comfortable. She declined his suggestion and went back home.

Rather than give up on herself and her situation, Dr. Parcells started to think about how she might heal herself, since the medical establishment had offered no hope. In those days, there were no books to read on the subject of alternative health and no alternative healthcare practitioners in the area where she lived. She was on her own. It was up to her to heal herself *if* that was even possible. She began to "listen" to her body. Realizing that "we are what we eat," she considered how she had been nourishing herself. She noticed that she craved green foods, in particular, and began eating leafy greens—as many as she could find. At that time of year, spinach was just about the only green available. It was practically all she ate for weeks on end. She ate it cooked as well as raw in fresh salads, and she drank plenty of spinach juice. It was as though she couldn't get enough of those greens.

In her beauty salon, where she continued to work despite her pain, she had installed one of the "modern" inventions of the time—a machine that invigorated the facial skin of her clients who were seeking beauty treatments. In order to administer the treatment, she strapped applicators onto her arms. When the machine was turned on, the applicators caused a vibration down her arms all the way to her fingers. Then she would massage the client's head and face with her hands. She later came to discover that it was the folic acid from the spinach in combination with the electromagnetic energy flowing through her body that encouraged the amazing transformation she would soon experience

She returned to the hospital in Denver six months later for a follow-up examination. Much to the astonishment of the doctor, the new x-rays showed an outline of re-formation taking place in the kidney. Plus her lungs had stopped hemorrhaging and her heart was less swollen. She was advised to keep doing what she was doing, and so she went back home and continued her self-treatment, which largely focused on eating the right foods and listening to her body. In less than a year, she had healed herself without drugs or medications of any kind.

Her "kitchen chemistry" experiments, as she called them, not only led to her miraculous recovery, but thrust her into an entirely new career in the field of nutrition. Listening to her many discoveries, I was in awe. She was at least fifty years ahead of her time. She talked a lot about the energetics of health, explaining that everything we do, eat, or drink affects us on a cellular level. She even predicted that people would be drinking bottled water someday as they wouldn't be able to get clean water from a tap. This was long before bottled water became the norm here in the United States. She also developed recipes for therapeutic bath formulas that are still used today with remarkable results. As 65 percent of body cleansing is done through our skin, the body's largest organ, Dr. Parcells designed her formulas to help pull out environmental chemicals, pesticides, heavy metals, and even harmful radiation.

She talked about the importance of ruling out parasites as the first step in helping someone who is chronically ill. "If someone has an overload of parasites," she said, "they're not going to be able to absorb nutrients or maintain health. Parasites are immunosuppressive, affecting one's overall energy." She advocated careful lab testing for parasites and developed two purging programs for ridding the body of them—further backing up all the information Ann Louise and I had gathered about the dangers of parasites.

Dr. Parcells also stressed the importance of maintaining the body's correct pH level—the acid-alkaline balance. Using the analogy of a plant and soil, she explained that if you periodically sprinkle salt around the base of a plant, over time you will eventually change the pH of the soil, and the plant might begin to die. You can reverse this by correcting the pH of the soil and, over time, the plant will begin to thrive again. If your lawn looks unhealthy and the grass is dying in patches, or if the plants in your garden aren't thriving, it's a good bet that the soil's pH balance is off. Depending on the missing minerals or nutrients, the problem may be corrected with fertilizer, lime, or nitrogen compound. The point is that a great looking lawn or healthy fruits and vegetables from the garden require healthy soil. It doesn't matter if you buy the best-looking tomato plant at the nursery, if you plant it in unhealthy soil, it will struggle. By the same token, our bodies must have the proper nutrients and pH balance to be healthy. It's not an overnight process, however, to change the composition of the soil or of your body. It takes time and persistence to get well. Prevention is much easier!

I told Dr. Parcells that I'd had cancer. She wasn't fazed at all. She said, "Cancer is nothing but a man-made word with fear dripping all over it." To her, it was simply the evidence of a body out of balance. At first we may not realize we're out of balance, she explained, but if left alone for too long, our bodies will get our attention with "disease." She believed that a diagnosis of cancer simply meant that you had another chance to get your body back in balance. The longer you delay, she warned, the sicker you'd get. It's all about figuring out *why* you're out of balance and then getting your body back in balance. Then the cancer can begin to heal.

When the body is going haywire from any degenerative disease, Dr. Parcells believed that you must get to the root cause—and, fortunately, there's a process for that. You first have to detoxify. Get rid of the toxins that are affecting your body's immune system or its ability to absorb nutrients. Toxins can include parasites, viruses, bacteria, radiation, heavy metals, contaminated water, irradiated food, and often the environment in which we live. The more toxicity you remove from your body, the stronger you'll be. It's like peeling away the layers of the onion and getting to the root. These are things we know about now, but fifty years ago, she was one of the few talking about them.

Dr. Parcells pointed out that the soil today isn't like the soil 100 years ago or even when she was a little girl. We're not getting the same quality of fruits and vegetables from our land than in times past. We haven't taken good care of our environment, nor have we properly restored the nutrients in the soil that have been depleted over time. We don't practice crop rotation as we should. We allow contamination of our water and soil. What we don't realize is what we do to our soil, we do to ourselves. Without proper soil, you simply can't grow healthy fruits and vegetables. That is why minerals and nutritional supplements are necessary in these modern times.

Dr. Parcells had a large teaching kitchen with several stoves, sinks, and counters where she lectured and taught others about the chemistry of foods. In her cooking classes, she stressed the importance of cleaning foods to remove impurities and restore their energetic value. I remember spending time with her one day, watching and learning what she did and how she did it. We were in her lab and it was lunchtime. "Come in the kitchen, honey, and let's have something to eat," she said. When we got to the kitchen, she filled up two bowls with beans and ham hocks that had been cooking in a crockpot.

"Doctor," I said. "I can't eat this. It has pork."

She responded in a kind, but firm voice, "Now, listen here. Yes, you can. You can eat pork. You can eat just about anything."

"But I haven't eaten meat in I don't know how many years!" I explained. "I'm on a strict macrobiotic diet." The truth was, I was thin. I had energy and felt good, but I had lost a lot of muscle mass from lack of protein over the past few years. Dr. Parcells looked me up and down and said, "Your color is not the best. You're not as vital as you should be. You're going to have to start eating meat again because if you don't, you're going to get sick again. If you stay on a healing diet too long without proper protein, you will get sick. Again, you can eat just about anything if you clean it up properly."

I wasn't sure if I was ready for this. I sat for a minute and looked at this healthy, vibrant woman who was well over one-hundred years old and thought about what she was saying. How many people did I know in the natural health field who had lived to be over one hundred and was as sharp as she was? How many had overcome sickness as she had? How many had studied and researched as much as she had? No one. Well, I ate that lunch, and let me tell you, it was so good! My body was craving meat. It had been over six years since I'd eaten anything like that. Looking back, I'm not sure where I'd be if she hadn't shown me that the diet that *got me well* was not the same diet that would *sustain me* for the long run.

I thought I would be following the macrobiotic diet for the rest of my life because that's what helped save my life. I came to understand that cancer grows in an acidic environment. The macrobiotic diet works so well because it not only helps to detoxify, but it helps the body become more alkaline in order to fight off illness. But once the illness is reversed, you have to build up your system, particularly the endocrine system—your glands. And that requires a different kind of diet according to Dr. Parcells. She added, "You show me a vegetarian, and I'll show you a person who dies before their time. They're not supporting their glands properly. You have to feed the body what it needs to support the glands properly." I'm not saying that she was 100-percent right and I don't know if I necessarily agreed with that statement, but it's what she said. It was certainly something to think about.

Dr. Parcells went on to explain her methods of cleaning and rejuvenating foods—meats, vegetables, and fruit. One was a technique she discovered in the 1960s while head of the Nutrition Department of Sierra States University. She would soak foods for specified amounts of time in a solution of sodium hypochlorite and water, giving them a thorough rinse afterward. The original *Parcells Oxygen Soak* is registered with the Smithsonian Institution. According to some of her students, it is recommended to use a $1/2$ teaspoon of regular Clorox® per one gallon of water. The other technique was her use of full spectrum light to restore food energy that was lost in production and transit. It also nullified the harmful effects of pesticide residue, heavy metals, and additives.

According to Dr. Parcells, the two most important ways to maintain health and longevity are the following:

1. Keep the body's pH balanced. Much like the pH level of soil must be correct in order to grow plants and vegetables, the chemistry of the body must have the correct pH to maintain health. Generally speaking, the body's pH level needs to be over 7.2 in order to heal. The cells and their energy are universal keys to health. Dr. Parcells believed that balancing your pH on a daily basis will keep away all forms of disease. She told me it was essential to keep my cancer from returning. There are many ways to measure your pH. One is with test strips that measure pH through saliva or urine. These can be found at most local drugstores or even ordered online.

2. Support the endocrine system. This network of glands that produce and release hormones, regulate many important body functions. Glands are the energy centers of the body, and our bodies are electromagnetically charged. She used the analogy of a car. Our glands are like a car's

alternator. If the alternator isn't functioning, the battery won't work and you won't be going anywhere. Likewise, if your glands aren't functioning properly, your body won't have the energy it needs to sustain itself.

Dr. Parcells stressed the importance of keeping glands in balance. This involves the body's *chakras*—seven energy centers that help regulate the body's processes, from organ function to the immune system to emotions. Each chakra is paired with a specific endocrine gland. The table below lists each chakra, the endocrine gland it is connected with, and the gland's function. Also listed are the organs affected by each chakra.

THE BODY'S SEVEN ENERGY CENTERS AND THE BODY PROCESSES THEY REGULATE			
CHAKRA	AFFECTED GLAND	GLAND FUNCTION	AFFECTED ORGAN
Root chakra (1st)	Reproductive glands (testes in men; ovaries in women)	Controls sexual development and secretes sex hormones.	Testes, kidneys, spine
Sacral chakra (2nd)	Adrenal glands	Regulates the immune system and metabolism.	Bladder, prostate, ovaries, kidneys, gall bladder, bowel, spleen
Solar Plexus chakra (3rd)	Pancreas	Regulates metabolism.	Intestines, pancreas, liver, bladder, stomach, upper spine
Heart chakra (4th)	Thymus gland	Regulates the immune system.	Heart, lungs
Throat chakra (5th)	Thyroid gland	Regulates body temperature and metabolism.	Bronchial tubes, vocal cords, respiratory system, all areas of the mouth, including tongue and esophagus
Third Eye chakra (6th)	Pituitary gland	Produces hormones and governs the function of the previous five glands; sometimes, the pineal gland is linked to the third eye chakra as well as to the crown chakra.	Eyes, pituitary and pineal glands, brain
Crown chakra (7th)	Pineal gland	Regulates biological cycles, including sleep.	Spinal cord and brain stem

Whenever one of our energy centers is thrown off balance, physical problems can manifest. Dr. Parcells explained the importance of feeding our glands the nutrients they need in order to perform their work. In addition, she felt the healing power of color is very influential in strengthening our chakras, and thus our glands and organs. She often said that the one tool for natural self-healing that she felt most important was color. She taught me that looking at light through a prism was another way to energize our chakras. In addition, she showed me how to place a prism over a glass or jar of water, set it in the sunlight, and let the sunshine energize the water. Drinking this water helps to energize any weak areas in the body.

The secret to health in a nutshell, she explained, is to clean your body from the ground up, rebuild, and maintain—and it's important to do it in that order. First, check for parasites and detoxify as needed. If glands are strong and pH on a cellular level is correct, then the body thinks it's younger than it really is. If your glands are weakened for a long period of time, your body thinks it's supposed to start dying. As we get older, we must take better care of our body, especially the glands. She explained that we're all going to die of something and our bodies will eventually wear out, but when it comes to dying before your time, it's because you haven't taken care of yourself. We can fool the body into thinking it's younger than it really is, simply by keeping it energized through proper nutrition, detoxification, elimination, and supplementation.

When I think about Dr. Parcells and the way she looked at things, I like to use the analogy of a car. Imagine you get one car to last your entire lifetime. That car better be built pretty dang well and it must be well maintained. If it has some weak parts (genetics), or some issues with certain parts, you still have to keep that car. So you'd better take care of it. Let's say that when you're young, you like to drive fast and brake hard. If that's the case, you're going to wear that car out and have issues sooner than someone who drives their car easy and treats it well. It's common to think you're invincible when you're young, and believe me, I was no exception. I abused my body. I ate the wrong foods, drank too much, and didn't protect my skin as I should have. Those who didn't make lifestyle changes for the better are more than likely paying the price today.

If you don't take good care of your car, there's a good chance you're going to have to replace some of its parts. And yes, like a car, you can replace body parts these days, but you can't, for example, replace your heart as easily as you can replace your car's water pump. Many of us have driven our bodies hard when we were young, and it can be a maintenance nightmare to restore them back to health. There's also a good chance that they may simply give out years before they should. On the other hand, those who have driven their bodies well, can maintain them for years and years. Heck, a vintage body, like a vintage car, is a thing of beauty!

I remember attending one of Dr. Parcells' seminars while we were in Albuquerque. There was a seventy-eight-year-old man in the class who complained about his advancing age and not feeling as good as he used to. She listened politely and then turned to him and said, "You're nothing but a young pup! You're not old, you just think you're old. You're only as old as you feel so if you feel old, then do something about it!"

Dr. Parcells was feisty and witty and loved to laugh at herself and her own jokes. She enjoyed telling stories, too. She drove her car to work every day until she was one-hundred years old. Someone mentioned to her, "Doctor, don't you think maybe you shouldn't drive anymore because of the liability issues?" She laughed and said, "I guess you're probably right." And she stopped driving as a matter of personal choice at age one-hundred.

When she was 104 years old, she started looking for a large piece of property where she could build a retreat for people who wanted to come and stay and study. She knew there was a lot of radiation in Albuquerque and the Santa Fe area, so she wanted to get away from that environment and be further up in the mountains. When she found a small ranch she wanted to buy, she went to the local bank for a loan. The banker was younger than she was, but not exactly the picture of health. He was carrying too much weight and his color wasn't good. He denied giving her the loan, saying, "Listen here, Dr. Parcells, at your age, we would be taking a big risk in loaning money to you." She looked at him, shook her finger and said, "You listen here, Sonny. You may think I'm old, but I'm going to tell you something right now. You're nothing but a walking time bomb waiting to explode and I'd be a lot more worried about myself if I were you!" And she walked out of that bank and never went back. She eventually got the land she wanted, but not from that bank.

Meeting and getting to know this marvelous woman was one of the highlights of my life. Her common sense, down to-earth-approach combined with her amazing experiments in the field of nutrition and energetics helped to turn my life around and put me on a lifelong course of learning and helping others with new insight and information. How could you not appreciate someone who defied a death sentence, healed herself, and lived to be 106?

Life is an experiment. We learn as we go along. No matter what we do, it's important that we don't ever give up! Just figure out why you're having problems, fix them, and get well. Make your body a fortress so that you can fight off illnesses. Remember that maintaining health is a never-ending process of checks and balances.

8

The Vitamin C Connection

"I believe that you can, by taking some simple and inexpensive measures, lead a longer life and extend your years of well-being. My most important recommendation is that you take vitamins every day in optimum amounts to supplement the vitamins that you receive in your food."
—Dr. Linus Pauling

When you charge like a bull into your own healing, willing to fight and do whatever it takes, I believe everything you need to get the job done will come to you. Thanks to *Cancer and Vitamin C*, the book by Dr. Linus Pauling that Mama brought me in the hospital, I learned about the miracles of this humble but powerful vitamin. I remember getting so excited when I read how patients with terminal cancer would take up to 10,000 milligrams (mg) of vitamin C every day and often experience a miraculous turnaround. I remember thinking that if vitamin C worked for those terminal cancer patients in Dr. Pauling's studies, why wouldn't it work for me, too?

The path in front of me was clear—after my escape from the hospital, I used the macrobiotic diet and lifestyle to change the way I lived my life and began taking vitamin C to further increase my odds of survival. When I first started out, I figured that if 10,000 mg a day was good, then 20,000 mg was even better, so that's what I took. The vitamin C was in tablet form and buffered with magnesium and lysine. The tablets were also timed-release, which meant they would enter my system slowly and be easier on my stomach in the long run. When taking large doses of vitamin C, I was warned that some people might experience loose stools, but it didn't have that effect on me. It's recommended that you take vitamin C until bowel tolerance and backing off until your bowels work normally. In other words, your body's tolerance level for vitamin C fluctuates depending on how much your body can withstand. You can't overdose—if you have too much too soon, the only negative effect you might get is loose stools. But that happens only when your body can't absorb any more vitamin C, and that is your cue that you've had enough. The good news is that once you get to bowel tolerance, the body's immune system has its best chance of kicking into gear.

I was getting off to a good start on the macrobiotic diet, the cornerstone of my cancer healing, but adding vitamin C gave me a lot more energy and seemed to noticeably strengthen my immune system. It wasn't long before I could really tell the difference. For the first time in many years, I wasn't getting sick with colds or flus. Even my seasonal allergies started to go away. I felt the vitamin C was working, so I stuck with it. I think that it makes sense to take enough vitamin C to make a difference. I've taken high doses for many years and never had any issues. Of course, before taking high dosages of vitamin C, it's important to consult your doctor or healthcare provider to be sure it is right for you.

Over the years, I have learned a lot of important information about vitamin C and a few other key nutrients, as well as the back story of the doctors, scientists, and researchers who brought this information to light. In this chapter, I want to share some of the noteworthy material I've learned.

A LANDMARK STUDY

Dr. Linus Pauling was an American chemist, biochemist, peace activist, author, and educator. For his scientific work, Pauling was awarded the Nobel Prize in Chemistry in 1954. For his peace activism, he was awarded the Nobel Peace Prize in 1962. He is one of four individuals to have won more than one Nobel Prize, the others being Marie Curie, John Bardeen, and Frederick Sanger. Of them, he is the only one awarded two unshared Nobel Prizes and one of two to be awarded the prize in different fields, the other being Marie Curie. Pauling published numerous books and hundreds of scientific papers. *New Scientist* called him one of the twenty greatest scientists of all time.

In the early 1990s, Dr. Pauling teamed up with physician/researcher Dr. Matthias Rath to do what turned out to be a landmark study on the effect of vitamin C on different forms of cancer. Born in 1955 in Stuttgart, Germany, Dr. Rath received his medical degree from Hamburg University

Medical School. In 1989, he was invited to begin working at the Linus Pauling Institute of Science and Medicine.

It might sound too good to be true that this simple, inexpensive vitamin, which can be bought over-the-counter at any drugstore, could be effective against such a baffling and resistant disease as cancer. However, according to the research of these doctors, it can stop the disease in its tracks.

The study, which spanned fifteen years, involved two groups. One group received a combination of vitamin C, L-lysine, L-proline, and EGCG (a green tea extract). The other group was put on a placebo. Research was conducted on more than two dozen cancer cell types, with results showing that the nutrient combination was effective in controlling cancer in many ways. It stopped the growth, the spread, the formation of new blood vessels in tumors (angiogenesis), and caused the natural death of cancer cells (apoptosis). At the end of the study, the researchers discovered that cancer was a collagen disease. That is, it spreads to the different tissues through the collagen.

COLLAGEN IS KEY

Collagen is the most abundant protein in the human body. More than 80 percent of the skin is composed of collagen, and it is the main component of ligaments and tendons. You could say that it is the "glue" that holds the body together. Cells are surrounded by collagen and connective tissue. Some types of collagen fibers, gram-for-gram, are stronger than steel. Even so, cancer cells contain an enzyme (nagalase) that can eat right through collagen. The amino acid L-lysine destroys this collagen-eating enzyme. High amounts of vitamin C strengthen the collagen so the cancer has a hard time penetrating and spreading. When cancer cells can't spread, they have difficulty surviving. *Metastasis*, the invasion of cancer cells into other organs and tissues, causes 90 percent of cancer deaths. According to the Pauling-Rath study, the simple micronutrient combination of vitamin C, the amino acids L-lysine and L-proline, and EGCG, a green tea extract, prevents metastasis. (See "The Rath Protocol" on page 84.) This nutrient combination was shown to block several cancer types—melanoma, cervical, ovarian, breast, prostate, testes, lung, kidney, pancreas, colon, bladder, osteosarcoma, fibrosarcoma, and synovial sarcoma—from invading the collagen layers.

The Rath Protocol

The micronutrient combination used in the fifteen-year landmark study led by Drs. Matthias Rath and Linus Pauling is detailed below. Study results showed it to be effective in stopping the spread of cancer cells through collagen, the means by which metastasis occurs.

- **Vitamin C** in its lipid-soluble form, *ascorbyl palmitate*, has been shown to be effective in eliminating abnormal cells in the body while protecting normal cells. Vitamin C is not produced by the human body.

  Chen, Q., Espey, M.G., et al. (2005) Pharmacological ascorbic acid concentrations selectively kill cancer cells: Action as a pro-drug to deliver hydrogen peroxide to tissues. *Proceedings of the National Academy of Sciences* 102(38): 13604–13609.

- **L-lysine** and **L-proline** are natural amino acids that are the building blocks of collagen and elastin fibers. L-lysine prevents digestion of collagen by blocking sites where enzymes attach, making this nutrient critical in preventing the destruction of connective tissue. Although L-proline is produced by the human body in limited quantities, L-lysine is not. The health of the connective tissue depends on optimal daily intake of these two key amino acids, as well as vitamin C.

  Rath, M., Pauling, L. (1992) Plasmin-induced proteolysis and the role of apoprotein(a), lysine, and synthetic lysine analogs. *Journal of Orthomolecular Med* 7: 17-23.) (Kikuchi, Y., Kizawa, I., et al. (986) The inhibitory effect of tranexamic acid on human ovarian carcinoma cell grown in vitro and in vivo. *Gynecol Oncol* 24(2): 183–188.

- **Epigallocatechin gallate** (EGCG) is an important compound of green tea. EGCG works at the cellular level to intervene against various cancers and suppress tumor growth.

  Dermeule, M., Brossard, M., et al. (2000) Matrix metalloproteinase inhibition by green tea catechins. *Biochim Biophys Acta* 1478(1): 51–60.) (Zhang, G., uira, Y., et al. (2000) Induction of apoptosis and cell cycle arrest in cancer cells by in vivo metabolites of teas. *Nutr Cancer* 38(2): 265–273.

Based on these impressive findings, I have made these supplements part of my daily regimen. For more information on this subject or for a customized program to fit your own specific needs, consult your healthcare practitioner. You can also contact the Dr. Rath Research Institute at www.drrathresearch.org for more information.

Humans are unable to manufacture vitamin C, and it's hard to get enough through fruits and vegetables. The body doesn't produce lysine either. To get enough of these nutrients to help in the fight against cancer, they have to be supplemented in highly absorbable forms. Because vitamin C is water soluble (it flushes out of your body through the urine), it needs to be taken more often or in a timed-release formula to be effective.

Vitamin C is usually supplemented orally in one of three forms: ascorbic acid, calcium ascorbate, or sodium ascorbate. It is one of the few nutrients that is extremely difficult to overdose on. That being said, you'll want to be sure you drink lots of water if you take megadoses (2,000 mg or more per day). But optimal hydration is important for good health in general, so you should never let your body get dehydrated. In general, it is recommended to drink one-half to one ounce of water for every pound of body weight. So if you weigh 120 pounds, you should drink 60 to 120 ounces of water each day.

INTRAVENOUS VITAMIN C THERAPY

If you have cancer, taking vitamin C intravenously is something to consider. Frederick R. Klenner, MD, a graduate of Duke University School of Medicine in 1936, was the originator of successful high-dose intravenous vitamin C therapy. He was the first to use it in viral diseases successfully, including polio. In an article written by Klenner that appeared in the *Journal of Applied Nutrition,* he wrote: "After vitamin C has entered cells infected by viruses, vitamin C 'proceeds to take up the protein coats being manufactured by the virus nucleic acid, thus preventing the assembly of new virus units.' Some infected cells expand, rupture, and die, but there are no virus particles available to enter and infect new cells. If a virus has invaded a cell, the vitamin C contributes to its breakdown."

Dr. Klenner successfully treated chicken pox, measles, mumps, tetanus, and polio with huge doses of the vitamin. He emphasized that small amounts do not work. He said, "If you want results, use adequate ascorbic acid." He considered a therapeutic level of daily vitamin C supplementation to be 350 mg per kg body weight (2.2 lbs. body weight), and he often recommended much larger amounts. Dr. Klenner found that the following conditions responded to extremely high-dose vitamin C therapy:

- Alcoholism
- Arthritis
- Atherosclerosis
- Bladder infections
- Burns and secondary infections
- Cancer, some types
- Chronic fatigue
- Complications from surgery
- Corneal ulcers

- Diabetes
- Encephalitis
- Glaucoma
- Heat stroke
- Heavy metal poisoning (mercury, lead)
- Hepatitis
- Herpes simplex virus
- Herpes zoster virus (shingles)
- High cholesterol

- Leukemia
- Mononucleosis
- Multiple sclerosis
- Pancreatitis
- Pneumonia
- Radiation burns
- Rocky Mountain spotted fever
- Ruptured intervertebral discs
- Schizophrenia
- Venomous bites

All of Dr. Klenner's papers are listed and summarized in the *Clinical Guide to the Use of Vitamin C* (ed. Lendon H. Smith, MD, Life Sciences Press, Tacoma, WA, 1988).

Dr. Ronald Hoffman of the Hoffman Center in New York City, a clinic that utilizes high-dose IV vitamin C drips as part of its progressive cancer treatment protocols, writes: "IV vitamin C, when administered by a trained, experienced physician, is safe and well-tolerated, even at doses as high as 100,000 mg (100 grams) per day. Proper blood tests must be done to ensure that it is well-tolerated, and the patient must be monitored. Doses must be gradually adjusted upward." Bypassing the body's digestive buffers allows intravenous vitamin C to spur the production of hydrogen peroxide deep within bodily tissues. And with the help of disease-fighting white blood cells, this "peroxide-mediated" vitamin C, as Dr. Hoffman puts it, performs unique and key functions in the targeting and eradication of cancer cells wherever they might be lurking in the body.

Even the National Cancer Institute (NCI) is on board with the science behind IV vitamin C therapy. It admits, based on laboratory studies, that vitamin C is capable of helping to slow the growth of cancer cells in the prostate, pancreas, liver, and colon. Both animal and human studies have also shown that IV vitamin C therapy can help block tumor growth and improve patient quality of life.

CANCER CELLS MISTAKE VITAMIN C FOR GLUCOSE

With the establishment of The Center for Healing Arts in 1975, Dr. Hugh Riordan routinely checked plasma vitamin C levels in chronically ill patients (plasma is the liquid part of the blood and lymphatic fluid). Interestingly, the cancer patients he was seeing had *very low* vitamin C reserves. This matched scientific literature documenting low vitamin C levels in cancer patients. Cancer cells thrive on glucose. According to Ron Hunninghake, M.D., Chief Medical Officer, Olive W. Garvey Center for Healing Arts: "Because the molecular shape of vitamin C is remarkably similar to glucose, cancer cells will actively transport vitamin C into themselves, possibly because they mistake it for glucose."

If large amounts of vitamin C are presented to cancer cells, large amounts will also be absorbed. In these unusually large concentrations, the antioxidant vitamin C will start behaving as a pro-oxidant as it interacts with the copper and iron within the cells. This chemical interaction produces small amounts of hydrogen peroxide, which will continue to build up until it eventually destroys the cancer cells from the inside out. This effectively makes high-dose IV vitamin C a non-toxic chemotherapeutic agent that can be given in conjunction with conventional cancer treatments.

To sum it up, based on the work of several vitamin C pioneers before him, Dr. Riordan was able to prove that vitamin C was selectively toxic to cancer cells if given intravenously in large doses.

THE HYDROGEN PEROXIDE CONNECTION

Cancer researchers have homed in on how high-dose vitamin C kills cancer cells without damaging normal cells. When vitamin C breaks down, it generates hydrogen peroxide. A study conducted at the University of Iowa Health Care shows that tumor cells with low levels of the enzyme catalase are much less capable of removing hydrogen peroxide than normal cells—making the cancer cells susceptible to death when exposed to high doses of vitamin C. Normal cells which contain much higher levels of catalase are able to remove hydrogen peroxide, keeping it at very low levels so it does not cause damage.

VITAMIN C AND DENTAL PROCEDURES

Hal A. Huggins, DDS, was an early adopter of the concept of integrative medicine and is considered the grandfather of the holistic dental movement. He is best known for his efforts in persuading the dental industry to stop using mercury in fillings, which he believed to be toxic and contributors to a number of health problems, including autoimmune diseases. He also believed that root canals, dental implants, and even cavitations (holes in the jawbone where bone or teeth are removed) can be deadly, as they harbor extremely toxic bacteria that may then infect other parts of your body.

In the 1990s cardiologist and noted author Thomas E. Levy, MD, JD, was asked to assist Dr. Huggins with a number of his patients, who were suffering from one or more serious health problems. Prior to sedating these health-challenged patients for the dental procedures they required, Dr. Huggins had Dr. Levy administer a specific protocol of intravenous vitamin C. As Dr. Levy writes in his book, *Curing the Incurable*, he was not familiar with such a practice, but was greatly impressed as patients showed marked improvement soon after the procedure. As a result of these impressive results, which Dr. Levy witnessed time and time again, his interest in vitamin C was greatly aroused. This prompted his intensive research on both the toxicity caused by certain dental work like mercury fillings and the ability of vitamin C to help resolve it.

The wide-ranging health benefits of vitamin C, including its role in effectively treating dental toxicity, most infections, and even heart disease and cancer, became the focus of Dr. Levy's career. He has written several books and countless articles on the subject. He wrote about his personal life-changing experience with Dr. Huggins in "The Clinical Impact of Vitamin C: My Personal Experience as a Physician." In the article, Dr. Levy shares how Dr. Huggins opened his eyes to a "wide array of clinical approaches to different diseases with hitherto unheard-of clinical results at his clinic in Colorado Springs," writing:

> I can honestly say that my first visit to his clinic began the most meaningful part of my medical education. Nothing has been the same since. My office, where I practiced adult cardiology, ended up being shuttered shortly after that first visit. And I have never looked back. . . . Seeing was believing, and I realized the entire way that I approached patient care simply had to change. I needed to learn

a lot more about the intravenous delivery of this molecule known as ascorbic acid, or ascorbate. I resolved to research this vitamin as completely as possible, learn the nuances of that research as best I could, and then proceed to spread the word on the application of this incredibly potent, inexpensive, and non-toxic substance. . . . Vitamin C is truly Nature's gift to health and healing.

Virtually all medical conditions are associated with increased oxidative stress, and the relief, or at least partial relief, of this oxidative stress with the vigorous administration of vitamin C and other quality antioxidants, will always help. The oxidative stress caused by disease and environmental toxins can deplete the body's level of vitamin C and other antioxidants. In serious illness, the body's reserve of vitamin C goes to zero because the rate at which the body regenerates it is far lower than the rate of depletion. This can require huge doses to bring it back to normal. Even if you are taking antibiotics or other prescription medicines, bringing your levels of vitamin C in your body back to normal, or temporarily supranormal, will virtually always result in profound benefits. The treatment is effective and, compared to the expense of conventional treatments, it is inexpensive. Few medicines and therapeutic interventions are more affordable than, and as non-toxic as, vitamin C. Even though something as extraordinarily beneficial as vitamin C might seem too good to be true, that's definitely not the case.

Ann Louise and I knew the late Dr. Huggins or "Doc" as he was affectionately known. He was a true master in the field of dentistry and a good friend. After removing my mercury amalgams, he prescribed mega doses of vitamin C. Seeing is believing. Doc determined that a patient's blood chemistry could be used as a method of monitoring the success of a patient's treatment, so I had same-day (24-hour) blood tests done before and after the procedure. I was astounded to discover that my blood chemistry results were much improved immediately afterward. Before the procedure, my white blood count was high, but less than 24 hours later, my blood count was back to normal and my immune system improved going forward. Bottom line—if you want to improve your health—and especially if you have cancer—you'll want to be sure your dental health is in tip-top shape.

VITAMIN C AND HEART DISEASE

Along with effectively treating a number of illnesses and other health conditions, vitamin C is able to improve the quality of arteries and help protect against heart disease. A few years ago, I was having some chest pains.
I had a calcium-score scan done because I thought my heart was involved.
It turned out that my symptoms were caused by exposure to mold in the
house we were renting at that time. Anyway, because initially I couldn't
figure out what was wrong, I flew to New York to see a cardiologist there
who was knowledgeable on the latest technology. As part of the exam,
I was sent to a special lab for a scan of my arteries. When the scan was
over, the technician said to me, "Can I have a talk with you?" As soon as I
heard those words, it was like PTSD (Post Traumatic Stress Disorder) set
in. Even with all the advances I had made over the years, I had a flashback
of the doctor telling me I had cancer. This time, however, I figured maybe
my arteries were clogged and in really bad shape.

When the technician asked, "What are you doing?" I immediately
tried to think of what I had been doing wrong. I told him I was trying to
eat healthy, exercise, and do all the right things. He said, "Well, whatever
you're doing, you'd better stick to it. Your arteries are like a baby's. In all
the years I've been doing this, I don't know if I've ever seen anything like
it." Upon hearing his words, I realized that I had jumped to the wrong
conclusion. That knot in my stomach disappeared. I knew then that along
with living a healthy lifestyle, taking mega-doses of vitamin C as a cancer
protocol was not only strengthening my immunity, it was also good for
my heart! To this day, similar tests continue to confirm the quality of my
arteries, and—considering my genetic predisposition to heart disease—I
see it as a double blessing.

I didn't know it at the time, but later learned that Dr. Matthias Rath,
who was involved with Dr. Pauling in the landmark study on vitamin C,
found that coronary heart disease, the cause of heart attacks and strokes,
is an early form of scurvy. Ascorbate deficiency is the precondition and a
common denominator of human cardiovascular disease. Dr. Rath's discovery revealed that the development of atherosclerotic deposits in the
arteries of the heart is triggered by a long-term deficiency of vitamin C in
the cells of the artery wall.

According to the Centers for Disease Control and Prevention (CDC),
for more than a decade, heart disease and cancer have claimed the first

and second spots respectively as the leading causes of death in the United States. Together, they are responsible for 46 percent of the nation's deaths. When you think about how a simple and relatively inexpensive supplement like vitamin C could dramatically help prevent or improve these two diseases, doesn't it make sense to at least try it?

HOPE FOR THE FUTURE

If vitamin C is so effective in fighting cancer, heart disease, and other health conditions, why don't more doctors prescribe it? Makes you wonder, doesn't it? Over the years, numerous health discoveries have been initially ignored by medical communities around the world.

Fresh citrus fruit, rich in vitamin C, was discovered as a cure for scurvy in the mid-1700s, yet this finding was ignored for nearly a century. Many thousands of people died in the meantime. Dr. Ignaz Semmelweis, the nineteenth-century Hungarian doctor who first advocated washing one's hands between patient procedures was ignored by the medical profession and died in disgrace for his belief. Toxic mercury was used as medicine well into the twentieth century. And so it goes . . .

Experiments and research on vitamin C continue to this day, so I am hopeful that soon it may get the respect it deserves. Dr. Linus Pauling and Dr. Matthias Rath are two of my heroes. They were ahead of their time, for sure. I believe their work and discoveries were one of the factors that helped to save my life. I decided many years ago that I wasn't going to wait for mainstream medicine to catch up with mavericks like these men. I appreciate the inspirational words of Dr. Rath, who said, "Fighting for a medical breakthrough against existing interests and dogmas is like sailing on the ocean. The wind that blows in your face becomes your compass." He added, "You don't have to be a university professor or Nobel Laureate; what counts is that heart attacks, strokes, cancer, and many other diseases will essentially be unknown in the future."

9

The Power of
a Positive Mindset

"If you realized how powerful your thoughts are,
you would never think a negative thought."
—PEACE PILGRIM

I know how hard it can be to stay positive when you're feeling down and out. I remember lying in the hospital bed following my experimental chemotherapy treatments and wondering if I would make it out alive. It was all I could do just to grit my teeth and prepare for the next day's treatment. Let's face it. When bad things happen in our lives, it's hard to focus on anything but the pain—whether physical, emotional, or a combination of both.

Believe it or not, there is a way out. It's called *hope.* I've thought a lot about that day when my desperate plea for help was answered by the gift of hope that three visitors brought me as I lay fighting for my life. The door to my hope was opened when I learned how others had fought and won their battles against cancer. Their methods were so different from anything I could have imagined at that time. Just the idea that there might be a way out of my crisis was enough to turn my thoughts up a notch, from desperate to hopeful. The more I learned and the more I focused on the possibility that there might be a way for my body to heal itself, the more excited I got. It was like climbing a ladder out of hell—one step at a time. I believe that a positive mindset is so important that I want to devote an entire chapter to it.

The cells in our body react to every thought and emotion that runs through our mind. It's been proven that negativity suppresses our immune system. Each thought we think acts as either soothing cellular nutrition or a poison dart that releases destructive toxins in our bodies. What we choose to think about plays a central role in creating and maintaining our health. Think about it. If you're driving in traffic and someone unexpectedly swerves out of their lane into yours, a cascade of emotions will flood your body as you feel the fear and react to the danger. Your body will immediately release certain hormones to prime it for a "fight or flight" response. Originally, this response involved early man's reaction upon coming face to face with a threatening situation, often a wild animal. His fear would cause him either to face the animal (fight) or run away (flight). In modern times, this response is the reaction to all types of fear, such as the fear of having a car accident as just described. Once you have reacted to the fear, whatever that fear may be, the crisis is over and your body will stop producing those hormones. If this "fight or flight" response happens occasionally, there won't be a problem. It's when you suffer from chronic, repeated stress, that the body can experience problems.

Our immune system gets fed up with constant high alerts. It's like calling the fire department every day and telling them your house is on fire. After weeks of repeated calls, they may stop coming or, at the very least, they may send only minimal help. Similarly, when the immune system is really needed, say to fight off an infection, it may no longer be in peak condition if it has been weakened by a barrage of chronic stress. And as you will see in the inset on page 95, researchers have shown this to be true.

My experience in fighting cancer led me to some unconventional treatments. The macrobiotic approach, for example, was a game changer for me, as it was the healing diet my body needed at that time. But just as that hospital psychotherapist had warned me, it took a lot of determination and hard work on my part. When I began the very strict protocol, no one else I personally knew was cooking or eating like I was. Keeping a positive mindset that what I was doing was beneficial to my health was difficult, but vital to my success. Just as important, I had to make a conscious effort to avoid negative people or situations. I couldn't afford to let myself be influenced by any naysayers.

The old saying, "misery loves company" is true and, conversely, positive people are attracted to positive people. Like attracts like. When I first met the folks at the Kushi Institute and found myself in the midst of all those encouraging people, I could feel the energy in the room and it immediately lifted my spirits. Haven't you noticed that when you enter a room full of people, you can sense whether they're upbeat or negative? When you're fighting cancer, I think that it's not only a good idea to surround yourself with positive people, it's absolutely vital to your health.

Stress Can Destroy Your Immune System

In the early 1980s, psychologist Janice Kiecolt-Glaser, PhD, and immunologist Ronald Glaser, PhD, of the Ohio State University College of Medicine, were intrigued by animal studies that linked stress and infection. For ten years, these pioneer researchers focused on this connection, using medical students as their study subjects. Among their findings, they discovered, through periodic blood samples, that the students' immunity went down every year under the simple stress of the three-day exam period. The test-takers had fewer natural killer cells, which fight tumors and viral infections. They almost stopped producing immunity-boosting gamma interferon and their infection-fighting T-cells responded only weakly to test-tube stimulation.

These findings opened the floodgates of research. Lab studies in which the subjects were stressed for just a few minutes showed them to experience a burst of "first responder" activity mixed with other signs of weakening. For stress of any significant duration—from a few days to a few months or years, as happens in real life—all aspects of immunity went downhill. The studies showed that long-term or chronic stress can ravage the immune system through too much wear and tear.

Further analysis also revealed that people who are older or even mildly depressed are more prone to stress-related immune changes. To serve as an example, a study by Lyanne McGuire, PhD, of Johns Hopkins School of Medicine that was done with Drs. Kiecolt-Glaser and Glaser, reported that even chronic, sub-clinical mild depression can suppress an older person's immune system. Participants in the study were in their early seventies and caring for someone with Alzheimer's disease. Those with chronic mild depression had weaker lymphocyte-T cell responses. As a follow up, the immune response was down even eighteen months later. It appeared that the key immune factor was duration, not severity, of depression. And in the case of the older caregivers, their depression and age meant a double-whammy for immunity.

While working at the Kushi Institute, I got to meet Dr. Patch Adams who helped transform the lives of many through his non-traditional practice. His prescription was laughter (or humor therapy if you prefer a more technical term). When you consider that laughter not only releases endorphins and other natural mood-elevating chemicals, but also improves the transfer of nutrients and oxygen to internal organs, it's no wonder that the old saying, "laughter is the best medicine" may very well be true.

Another technique I frequently used was visualization. Many athletes practice this to improve their performance. Visualization is simply a mental exercise in focusing your thoughts. You create images in your mind of having or doing whatever it is that you want in as much detail as possible. You then repeat these images over and over again, daily. It's a way to use your imagination to see yourself being successful in whatever goal you may have. It wasn't always easy to get the negative thoughts out of my head at times, but I would try anyway.

Whenever I had some time to myself, I would practice visualizing a healthy body. When I would go for walks, I would do my deep breathing, holding the oxygen in my lungs as long as I could, then release. I would picture the oxygen entering my body and destroying the cancer cells. When I would eat my meals, chewing my food 180 times and turning the food into liquid, I would picture every cell in my body absorbing the nutrients they needed to support my ability to fight off the cancer cells. I was starving the cancer cells by eliminating sugar, their food source, and strengthening my fighter cells by giving them the nutrition, vitamin C, and the oxygen they needed. I imagined there was a war going on inside my body, and I was arming the good guys to beat up the bad guys.

There have been several times in my life when I just needed to get away and spend some time alone. I would often choose to go where I wouldn't be influenced by anyone or anything but could spend time just getting in touch with a Higher Power. I did this when I packed up my things and spent a week alone in the mountains. Just being out in nature is in itself very healing. Hiking up a mountain made me feel strong and invincible. I wanted to prove to myself that I had what it would take to get well. When I made the decision to run eighteen miles, I had very little energy and I was still weak from surgery. But I *knew* that if I could accomplish that, I could do anything. I needed to strengthen my will so that my fighting spirit would kick in . . . and it worked.

A Story of Visualization and Positive Thinking

David Seidler, who won the Oscar for Best Original Screenplay for *The King's Speech*, was a stutterer just like King George VI, whose battle with the speech disorder is portrayed in the film. Seidler also suffered from cancer, just like the king. But unlike "His Majesty," Seidler survived the cancer. He said he did so because he used the same vivid imagination he employed to write his award-winning script. He said he visualized his cancer away. "I know it sounds awfully Southern California and woo-woo," he admits when describing the visualization techniques he used when diagnosed with bladder cancer six years earlier. "But that's what happened."

"When I was first diagnosed, I was rather upset, of course," Seidler said. "After three or four days of producing a lot of mucus and salty tears, I knew prolonged grief was bad for the autoimmune system, and the autoimmune system was the only buddy I had in fighting cancer."

After consulting with California urologist Dr. Dino DeConcini, Seidler decided not to have chemotherapy or have all or part of his bladder removed—common treatments for bladder cancer. Instead, he opted for limited surgery to remove just the cancer itself, and he took supplements to enhance his immune system. Despite his best efforts, the cancer came back within months. Seidler was forced to rethink his decision not to have chemotherapy or bladder surgery.

As his doctor booked an appointment for surgery two weeks later, Seidler commiserated with his soon-to-be-ex-wife, and it was a comment from her that gave him the idea to try to visualize his cancer disappearing. "She said, 'Well, what happens if in two weeks they go in and there's no cancer?'" He said, "I thought to myself that's the dumbest thing I've ever heard. This woman's in total denial." But later, reflecting upon her comments, Seidler thought she might be on to something—perhaps it would be possible for his cancer to just disappear while he waited for surgery. Figuring he had nothing to lose, for the next two weeks he imagined a clean bladder.

"I spent hours visualizing a nice, cream-colored unblemished bladder lining, and then I went in for the operation, and a week later, the doctor called me and his voice was very strange," Seidler remembers. "He said, 'I don't know how to explain it, but there's no cancer there.'" He said the doctor was so confounded he sent the tissue from the pre-surgical biopsy to four different labs, and all confirmed it was non-cancerous.

The doctor couldn't explain how it had happened, but Seidler could. He said he believed the supplements and visualizations were behind what his doctor called a "spontaneous remission." Plus, he believed a change in his way of thinking was also key. He stopped feeling sorry for himself because of both his cancer and his impending divorce. "I was very grief stricken," he remembers. "It was a thirty-year marriage, and in my grief, I could tell I was getting sicker. I decided to just change my head around."

While Seidler admitted that his unorthodox recovery techniques sounded "woo-woo" to some ears, they sounded "like science" to Dr. Christiane Northrup, a best-selling author, who has written extensively on the mind-body connection. "This doesn't sound woo-woo to me," she said. "The mind has the power to heal." By moving himself "from fear and abject terror into action," she believes Seidler changed his body's chemistry. "Fear increases cortisol and epinephrine in the body, which over time lower immunity." She believes that levels of these two stress hormones lead to cellular inflammation, which is the way cancer begins. Whether you're convinced of the effects of visualization or not, Northrup believes there's no harm in trying.

There is no definitive guide to visualization, but Dr. Bernie Siegel, retired clinical assistant professor of surgery at Yale Medical School and author of *Love, Medicine & Miracles*, who's instructed his patients in imaging for many years, has a few suggestions. First, he says to draw a picture of four things: yourself, your health problem, your treatment, and your body eliminating your problem. These pictures might tell you what sort of imagery would work best for you. For example, when one of Siegel's patients drew her disease as ten cancer cells next to one white blood cell, he suggested she visualize her body making more white blood cells.

Taking action through visualization can prove to be an important step in the fight against cancer or any health condition. It is an effort that can elicit hope. And according to Dr. Northrup, "Hope is actually a biochemical reaction in the body." And hope is a true gift that can produce positive results.

There's no doubt that a diagnosis of cancer can strike fear in your heart. The very word stirs up all sorts of emotions. And it's unrealistic to think you can be in control of your emotions all the time. Your attitude and mood can change from day to day, and even from hour to hour. You may feel good one day and terrible the next. There are also multiple ways for the body to heal. But if you can believe with all your heart that the method of treatment you choose will help you heal, and if you take great care to surround yourself with positive people and think positive thoughts, your body will respond by releasing the healing hormones and chemicals that you need.

Cancer, like any other serious condition, is not something to take lightly. You have to keep yourself as physically and mentally strong as possible. In my opinion, at least 50 percent of the work of healing is done in the mind. If the mind can heal the body, but the body cannot heal the mind, then the mind must be stronger than the body. The mind has to have a strong will, a sense of "if it doesn't work for me, it won't work for anyone else." Whether you're weak, strong, big, or small, you need that mentality. You need a powerful positive mindset. You have to let go of the past and envision a better future.

At some point in our lives, we've all been beaten up, knocked around, and kicked. We've had our share of ups and downs through relationships, sicknesses, and just living in this world. But sitting around dwelling on past mistakes will put you six feet under in no time. Do yourself a favor and cultivate a positive mindset. Surround yourself with positive people, read inspirational books, learn about how other people have successfully battled cancer, find your door to hope. Your body will thank you by shutting off the release of poisonous chemicals and hormones. Instead it will release a cascade of healing chemicals and hormones, strengthening your immune system so that you can better fight whatever comes your way.

Change can start in the mind. Healing can start with your thoughts. The mind is one of the biggest game changers when it comes to health and beating a fatal diagnosis. I am convinced of that.

10

Fight Like Your Life Depends Upon It

"You just can't beat the person who won't give up."
—BABE RUTH

To have a fighting chance against aggressive forms of cancer, you have to get serious . . . and I mean fast. Clearly, I understand how devastating being told you have cancer can be. Unfortunately, too many of us either freeze in place and let others choose the treatment options offered without asking questions, or worse, we accept what we believe is our fate and do nothing. While I initially chose the treatments that were offered to me, I knew that I needed to take back some level of control over my body. I came to realize that I needed to be more than a cancer victim. I began to see cancer as my enemy and that I needed to stockpile every weapon I could find to fight it.

When I first started dealing with my illness, I didn't know a hill of beans about what to do, and there weren't a lot of options available that I was aware of. But thank God for the information that was handed to me. At first, the path I chose seemed to come to me in pieces like a puzzle. But as you have read in the previous chapters, as the pieces fell into place, it created a roadmap—one that included a number of paths that led me to where I am now. In this chapter, I will be sharing information about those paths—the macrobiotic diet and lifestyle, vitamin C therapy, daily exercise, meditation, and more—and why I believe they worked for me. Keep in mind that this was my own personal roadmap in the fight against stage IV melanoma. Your search may lead you on a journey with different paths from mine.

THE MACROBIOTIC DIET

Pros: Very healing-oriented diet, restores proper gut flora, helps to restore homeostasis and proper alkalinity, and is very detoxifying.

Cons: Restrictive, time consuming, and must be properly implemented for best results.

People diet for different reasons. Personally, I benefited from the macrobiotic diet in my fight against cancer. In fact, when I look back, there is no doubt in my mind that it helped to save my life. Yes, cooking and preparing macrobiotic meals can take a lot of time and effort, but when done correctly, the diet can be enormously helpful. I went from eating a standard American diet to eating in a whole new way, and *it turned my life around.* Was it worth it? You betcha! So . . . what are the basics of the macrobiotic diet? What follows is a list of the recommended foods, followed by information on the cooking and preparation methods used for this diet.

Macrobiotic Foods

The following foods are recommended on the standard macrobiotic diet. It should be noted that for those with certain health conditions, like cancer, the diet is limited, more medicinal. Those who are healthy can eat a wider selection of these foods.

- **Whole grains.** Organically grown, non-GMO whole grains are the staple of a macrobiotic meal and make up 50 to 60 percent of the diet. Whole grains include brown rice, millet, barley, whole wheat, oats, rye, buckwheat, corn, sorghum, wild rice, amaranth, and quinoa.

- **Healing soups.** One to two small bowls of soup make up about 5 to 10 percent of the daily food intake. The broth is frequently made with miso and flavored with wheat-free tamari soy sauce. Several varieties of land and sea vegetables (listed below) may be added during cooking.

- **Organically grown vegetables.** Either cooked or raw, veggies make up at least 25 to 30 percent of the daily diet. A large amount of leafy greens, such as kale, collard greens, daikon greens, lettuce, turnip greens, mustard greens, bok choy, and watercress, are recommended. The chlorophyll they provide helps to detoxify. Other recommended vegetables include broccoli, cauliflower, cabbage, Chinese cabbage, carrots, celery, cucumbers, burdock, daikon radish, leeks, red and yellow onions, scallions, chives, parsley, and summer and winter squash. Those not recommended for regular use include beets, spinach, zucchini, and the nightshade vegetables: tomatoes, red and green bell peppers, potatoes, and eggplant.

- **Beans and bean products (non-GMO).** Lower-fat adzuki beans, lentils, chickpeas, and split peas make up about 10 percent of meals on a regular basis. Fermented soybean products, such as tempeh, tofu and natto, may be added.

- **Sea vegetables.** Rich in vitamins and minerals, sea vegetables are eaten daily in small amounts—no more than 5 percent. Common varieties including kombu, wakame, nori, dulse, and arame. They may be included in soups, cooked with vegetables or beans, or prepared as a side dish. As a side dish, they are usually seasoned with a moderate amount of wheat-free tamari soy sauce, sea salt, or brown rice vinegar.

  Note: *Hijiki is not included in this list as it has been shown to include high amounts of arsenic.*

- **Fish (wild).** For those in good health on a non-restricted diet, a small amount of certain wild-caught fish may be eaten a few times a week. White-meat fish generally contain less fat than red-meat or blue-skin varieties, and saltwater fish usually contain fewer pollutants than freshwater types. To help detoxify the body from the effects of fish, a small amount of grated daikon, horseradish, fresh ginger, or mustard is usually added to the meal as a condiment.

  Note: *Animal foods, including meat, poultry, eggs, and dairy are avoided except in infrequent cases when it may be recommended temporarily for medicinal purposes.*

- **Fermented foods.** Fermentation is an age-old food preservation process that also adds to the nutrient content of food. Almost any vegetable can be fermented, which makes them high in probiotics (friendly bacteria) for a healthy gut. In the macrobiotic diet, a small amount of homemade pickles is eaten each day to aid in the digestion of grains and vegetables. Traditionally, fermented pickles are made with a variety of root and round vegetables, such as daikon radish, turnips, cabbage, carrots, and cauliflower. The vegetables are aged in sea salt, rice or wheat bran, tamari soy sauce, umeboshi plums, shiso leaves, or miso. Keep in mind that all fermented foods must be unpasteurized. When buying fermented vegetables, look for the words "raw, unpasteurized" on product labels.

- **Seeds and nuts.** Lightly roasted organic sesame seeds, sunflower seeds, and almonds that can be seasoned with wheat-free tamari soy sauce or sea salt can be enjoyed as occasional snacks. Organic nuts and seeds are a healthy snack and a good source of protein and healthy fats that can be added to salads and a wide variety of other dishes.

- **Fruits.** Organically grown fruit may be eaten by those in good health a few times a week, preferably cooked or naturally dried, provided the fruit is grown in the local climate zone. When choosing fruit, it is best to choose only the lowest glycemic fruits. Raw fruit can also be consumed in moderate volume during its growing season. Most temperate-climate fruits, such as apples, pears, peaches, apricots, grapes, berries, and melons, are suitable for occasional use. Tropical fruits (with the exception of lemons) such as grapefruit, pineapple, and mango are not recommended. Fruit is not generally recommended for those with cancer, as any sugar in the diet feeds cancer.

- **Desserts.** For those who are in good health, desserts may be eaten in moderation two or three times a week. They are not recommended for those whose health is compromised. Common desserts on this diet include macrobiotic-approved cookies, puddings, cakes, pies, and other sweet dishes. Foods such as apples, fall and winter squash, parsnips, adzuki beans, or dried fruit can often be incorporated in recipes as natural sweeteners. For stronger sweetness, a natural grain-based sweetener, such as rice syrup, barley malt, or amazake, may be used.

- **Seasonings.** Organic brown rice vinegar, sweet brown rice vinegar, umeboshi vinegar, umeboshi plums, miso, soy sauce, and grated gingerroot are common seasonings for macrobiotic dishes. For sauces and gravies, kuzu root powder and arrowroot flour are acceptable thickeners. Sliced scallions, chives, parsley sprigs, nori squares or strips, and fresh grated gingerroot are common garnishes.

- **Condiments.** Gomashio (roasted ground sesame seeds and salt), roasted seaweed powders, umeboshi plums, and tekka (finely ground granules of dried root vegetables and miso) are among the popular condiments used in the macrobiotic diet.

- **Cooking oils.** All oils should be unrefined and GMO-free. For daily cooking, dark or light sesame oil is recommended. Safflower oil, olive oil, and walnut oil are acceptable for occasional use.

- **Beverages.** Drinks include spring or well water (at room temperature), bancha twig tea (kukicha), and grain-based teas like roasted barley tea and roasted brown rice tea. Grain coffee, umeboshi tea, dandelion root tea are taken occasionally. For those in good health, the following may be enjoyed less frequently: green tea, fruit juice, vegetable juice, soymilk, beer, wine, sake, and other grain, bean, vegetable, and herbal beverages.

This list of macrobiotic foods is based on a traditional Japanese diet. It was one of the keys to understanding why the Japanese had so few diseases that were common to those eating a standard western diet. Of course, with the introduction of fast foods and western-style meals in Japan, the Japanese are now suffering from many health disorders.

Harness the Power of Taste to Your Advantage

Different organs in the body are stimulated by different tastes. Sweet, sour, bitter, salty, and pungent—each stimulates a different organ. The macrobiotic diet, when done properly, will provide a variety of flavors that help to stimulate all body organs.

According to the macrobiotic philosophy:

Bitter. Bitter foods are thought to stimulate the heart and small intestine.

Salty. Salty food is thought to influence the kidneys and bladder.

Sweet. Sweet food is thought to influence the pancreas, spleen, and stomach.

Sour. Sour tasting food is thought to influence the liver and gall bladder.

Pungent. Pungent foods are said to beneficial to the lungs and colon, and they have been known to stimulate blood circulation.

Macrobiotic Cooking Methods

According to the macrobiotic way, cooking food should be done over a gas flame or, if convenient, a wood-burning fire. Avoid electric stoves if possible. This is because according to macrobiotic principles, the type of cooking has a direct impact on the food itself and the energy it produces. Fire imparts energy, vitalizing the human body physically, mentally, and spiritually. Cooking over fire results in food that is energized, more healing. The most common macrobiotic cooking techniques include pressure cooking, steaming, boiling, sautéing, and occasionally baking.

When I began my journey back to health, I cooked all of my meals myself. It was important for me to put effort and energy into my healing whenever I could. Cooking was part of my going to war, going to battle. It was about loving myself enough to take care of and nourish myself back to health. I will tell you this, cooking my meals took a lot of work, effort, time, and energy. But it was certainly worth it. I believe that food can pick up the energy of the person preparing it. I felt that I put good energy into the food I prepared by cooking with intention. For me, how you cook is just as important as what you cook.

How This Diet Affects a Healthy Gut

To understand the health benefits of the macrobiotic diet, it is important to know what is going on in your gut. The fact is that 70 to 80 percent of your immune system is situated in your digestive tract. And a healthy digestive tract relies on friendly bacteria and other microbes. Unfortunately, today's modern lifestyle can and does cause the disruption of a healthy gut through such factors as daily stress, the overuse of antibiotics, and a typical American diet that is high in sugar and high-glycemic foods, which can spike your blood sugar levels.

When the macrobiotic diet is followed correctly, the gut will flourish with good bacteria. Fermented foods, like sauerkraut, miso, kimchi, and natto, are recommended on the diet. The fermentation process for these foods creates probiotics—live beneficial bacteria—that help fortify the digestive tract. Along with being tasty, fermented foods are effective weapons in the fight against a compromised immune system.

Prebiotics are the fiber, the non-digestible part of foods like the skin of apples, the woody stems of celery, and the oat hulls in oatmeal.

Prebiotic fiber goes through the small intestine undigested and is fermented when it reaches the large intestine. It helps increase the beneficial bacteria in the gut.

Through my years of working in the health field, I've seen a lot of people, even kids, who were dealing with a variety of health issues, including rashes and allergies, and who were sick practically all the time. In my personal opinion, I believe that their bodies had too much toxicity and they didn't have enough good bacteria in their systems. When we eat the right foods in the right way, I believe it's entirely possible to fortify and strengthen our immune system so that we can live longer, healthier lives.

How the Macrobiotic Diet Affects pH Levels

Our bodies are meant to have a proper acid-alkaline balance. This balance is measured by the pH scale, which ranges from 1 to 14. The number 1 indicates most acidic while 14 is most alkaline. The normal range should fall between 7.35 and 7.45. (See "What's Your pH Level?" below.)

What's Your pH Level?

You can discover your pH level through your saliva or urine. This is done with the help of pH sticks or strips that you can purchase at most drugstores or pharmacies. The pH scale ranges from 1 to 14 with 7 being neutral. Values above 7 are alkaline, and below 7 are acidic. A normal pH range is from 7.35 to 7.45.

It is best to take your reading first thing in the morning before you eat or drink anything (except water) and before you clean your teeth. Try taking a reading every morning for a week to see the overall state of your saliva. If your readings are below 7 you are currently acidic. If your readings are between 7 and 7.5 you are what is considered healthily alkaline.

Many people tend to be too acidic, which is caused by too much sugar and animal food and not enough fiber. The goal is to become more alkaline. This can be done through diet as well as emotional well-being. Cancer has a hard time living in an alkaline environment. As it turns out, the macrobiotic diet is very alkalizing. It eliminates sugar (one of the biggest offenders) and fills the body with properly balanced nutrition. A little-known side-effect of sugar is its negative effect on the body's pH, resulting in a cascade of physical problems that can lead to chronic disease. Cancer thrives on sugar. If you have cancer, you'll want to be careful to avoid it in any form.

How the Macrobiotic Diet Keeps You Regular

The macrobiotic diet is also very good for elimination. From my point of view, if you're not having a bowel movement after pretty much each meal, you're not able to adequately eliminate all the toxins you should be getting rid of. Here's the scoop on poop: the faster food is digested, the less waste it leaves behind. The less waste left behind, the easier the digestion process. The easier the digestive process, the healthier you'll be!

If your body is on toxic overload, it will likely affect your immune system or your ability to absorb nutrients. You must get rid of the toxins, which, you will remember, can include parasites, viruses, harmful bacteria, radiation, heavy metals, pesticides, contaminated water, irradiated food, and even detrimental factors in our environment. The faster you get rid of these toxins, the less your body will have to work to fend them off. It allows your body to better defend your immune system. When I began following the macrobiotic diet, I had never eliminated so easily and regularly. Remember, the digestive tract is a two-way street. Feed it what it needs to maintain an abundance of healthy flora and give it what it needs to "take out the trash." The macrobiotic diet does both!

Proper chewing is another way in which this diet aids in both eliminating toxins and maximizing a food's nutritional benefits. At the start of my macrobiotic journey, I was somewhat thrown off by the amount of times I was supposed to chew my food—fifty times per mouthful! Normally, I would just gulp down whatever it was I was eating. However, as I purposely practiced chewing, I discovered that it allowed me to relax as I focused on the number of chews I needed before swallowing. I soon discovered that there was more to this than I first realized. When you chew food, you release saliva, which is rich in the enzyme *amylase*—an enzyme which starts the process of breaking down carbohydrates. With each chomp, your glands secrete more saliva and, therefore, more enzymes fill your mouth As the macrobiotic diet is higher in grains than most diets, these enzymes are important in breaking down the carbs. If you don't thoroughly chew your food, the amylase doesn't get a chance to do its job the way it should. Large food particles may not get broken down properly in your gut. Instead, they may enter your bloodstream where they can create a lot of havoc.

Although chewing each mouthful a minimum of fifty times is recommended on this diet, I figured I'd do better! So I made it my practice to chew each mouthful 180 times until it turned into liquid. While chewing, I focused on tasting what I was eating. I started to taste flavors I had never tasted before, and let me tell you, food never tasted so good! When you chew that much, it brings out the natural sweetness of many foods. It is amazing how vegetables can taste so sweet and flavorful. My desire for sugar simply disappeared. The very act of eating became a meditation for me. I enjoyed it so much that there were times I preferred to eat alone just so I could enjoy the experience uninterrupted.

I'm not saying that you need to chew as much as I did, but slowing down and chewing your food thoroughly will help your body digest the nutrients better than if you gulp down your food. Bottom line, the macrobiotic diet was a Godsend for me. I realize not everyone has the willpower or motivation to stick with it, but I'm glad I did. It was the healing diet that I needed at the time.

THE MACROBIOTIC LIFESTYLE

While the macrobiotic diet was the cornerstone of my healing process, following the macrobiotic lifestyle was equally important in restoring my body's balance and health. It is a lifestyle designed to create a connection between our diet, health, and environment. Through it, I learned the importance of community and of being around like-minded people. I learned to slow down, chill out, and to be intentional in everything I did. The macrobiotic lifestyle not only helped me physically and mentally, but strengthened me on an emotional level, too.

I learned the importance of wearing non-synthetic clothing, sleeping under non-synthetic sheets and blankets, and choosing all-natural fabrics instead. Through deep breathing techniques, Dōln exercises, yoga-type stretching (which make the body more flexible), and intentional visualization, I became my own healer. It was a powerful experience, one I'm glad

I embraced. It also opened my eyes to many other modalities as I searched for even more ways to heal my body.

The more I learned about how to heal my body, the more excited I became. Many of the principles were easy to adopt into my new lifestyle as I fought my way back to good health. And as I started seeing results and continued to gain in strength and vigor, I knew I was on the right track.

TAKING VITAMIN C

As mentioned in Chapter 8, I consider vitamin C to be vitally important. I've taken large doses of vitamin C supplements for over thirty-three years with great results. I can't even imagine a time when I would stop taking it! Our bodies don't make vitamin C naturally, so we have to get it from either food or supplements.

I can't say how much vitamin C is the right amount for anyone else, but I think that if you have cancer, it makes sense to be sure you're getting enough to make a difference. In all the years I've taken high doses, I've never had any issues. Studies have shown that vitamin C not only strengthens your immune system, it can kill cancer cells and block the growth of tumors.

One thing I haven't tried is high-dose intravenous (IV) vitamin C therapy. But if I were to be diagnosed with cancer today, I certainly would consider it. When taken by IV, vitamin C can reach much higher levels in the blood than when the same amount is taken by mouth.

There are certain situations in which high-dose vitamin C is not recommended. It is important to consult your healthcare practitioner before starting any vitamin or supplement regimen.

EXERCISING DAILY

Walking every day was part of my healing regimen and I really looked forward to it. Without a walk, I felt like I had missed a meal—it was that important to me. I didn't feel that I needed to burn myself out or beat myself up with overly strenuous exercise as I had done in the past. Instead, I learned it was better to relax and be gentle on my body. Healing takes a lot of energy, so I knew that it wasn't the time for a lot of strenuous exercise. Prior to getting diagnosed with cancer, I had spent a lot of days in the gym, but no longer did I feel that it was the ideal environment.

Instead, I headed outdoors—every day, all seasons—no matter what the temperature or weather condition. Being out in nature and seeing and experiencing the different seasons, was also helpful in stimulating both my sense of well-being and my lymphatic system.

If there is one system that directly impacts our immunity it is the lymphatic system. Considered a secondary circulatory system, the lymphatic system is a primary detoxication system. It rids the body of toxic waste, bacteria, heavy metals, and excess fat. It is the liver's partner in waste removal. Unlike blood, which is pumped by the heart, the lymphatic fluid has no pump. Instead, what moves the lymph through its many ducts and channels is exercise. To make it circulate, you have to pump it through movement.

The vessels in the lymphatic system branch throughout the body like the arteries and veins that carry blood. The lymph contains a high number of lymphocytes, a type of white blood cell that fights infection and destroys damaged or abnormal cells, including cancer cells if they are present. To this day, I'm handicapped by the lymph surgery I had, but I've worked hard to never let it stop me. Thankfully, I no longer have to use the lymph pump. By getting regular, daily exercise and following a healthy diet regimen, I have been able to put it away for good.

Deep breathing exercises during my walks were also extremely beneficial to me. Our bodies are meant to walk, breathe, and experience nature. I believe that hiking on trails and walking on this earth are important to my health. My best advice when walking is to choose a place that's far from the busy streets with their toxic exhaust fumes from cars and trucks. After all, we're trying to get rid of toxins, not take in more!

Shiatsu and Other Forms of Massage

Talk about waking the body up! Shiatsu and massage are very beneficial in simulating energy through the body. According to Eastern philosophy, this type of therapy stimulates our energy meridians. I did it as often as I could. All in all, shiatsu and massage have been very healing for my body.

In the Japanese language, shiatsu means "finger pressure". Shiatsu techniques include massages with fingers, thumbs, feet and palms; assisted stretching; and joint manipulation and mobilization. To examine a patient, a shiatsu practitioner uses palpation and sometimes pulse diagnosis. Shiatsu practitioners use their fingers, the palms of their hands, and even their elbows or feet. This type of therapy is beneficial in stimulating energy through the body. It's considered a type of complementary therapy—aimed to treat the whole person, not just the symptoms of disease. If you don't have access to a skilled shiatsu practitioner, take advantage of any therapeutical massage. All in all, I find shiatsu and other forms of massage to be very healing for my body.

Earthing / Grounding

I've always loved walking barefoot and sleeping on the earth. I often slept outdoors in my pup tent in all kinds of weather. I remember reading about how Native Americans considered contact with the earth to be highly beneficial. According to Ota Kte (Luther Standing Bear), Lakota Sioux writer, educator, and tribal leader: "The old people came literally to love the soil. They sat on the ground with the feeling of being close to a mothering power. It was good for the skin to touch the Earth, and the old people liked to remove their moccasins and walk with their bare feet on the sacred Earth. The soil was soothing, strengthening, cleansing, and healing."

Clint Ober, the author of *Earthing* and a former cable television executive asked a really great question about grounding: "If it is so critically important to television signals and any other sensitive electronics, would 'grounding' the human body, also a sensitive and complex electrical system, have similar beneficial effects?". He had been sitting on a park bench one day, when he noticed that many people were walking around in rubber soled shoes. Before modern times, people spent the majority of their time "grounded," walking barefoot and sleeping in caves. Based on his understanding of how cable wires must be grounded and shielded, he wondered if the rubber soled shoes were acting as an insulator from the natural healing energy of the Earth. If so, could it be affecting people's health?

Experimenting first on himself, Clint designed a conductive system for his bed, using metallic duct tape connected by wire to a grounding rod he planted in the soil outside. In this way, he could be in contact with the Earth's energy, simulating being barefoot outdoors. To his surprise, he found that such contact not only prompted sleep, but significantly reduced the chronic pain he had been experiencing. In 2000, he organized a group experiment to further test the results of this technique which he called "earthing". The results were impressive:

- 85 percent fell asleep faster.

- 93 percent reported sleeping better throughout the night.

- 100 percent reported waking, being and feeling more rested.

- 82 percent experienced a significant reduction in muscle stiffness.

- 74 percent experienced the elimination of/or a reduction of chronic back and joint pain.

- 78 percent reported improved general health.

In addition, several subjects in the study also reported experiencing significant relief from asthmatic and respiratory conditions, rheumatoid arthritis, PMS, sleep apnea, and hypertension.

Today there is a lot of information available that helps explain the science behind why it is so healthy for the body to be "grounded" as often as possible. We now know that the earth's surface is brimming with free electrons. Through a process known as *electron* transfer, the body readily absorbs the electrons when it comes into contact with them, whether by walking barefoot or by some other means of direct connection. The effects of this electron transfer and its impact on healing, and overall health is both shocking and impressive. A study published in the 2013 issue of the "Journal of Alternative and Complementary Medicine" showed that "grounding appears to be one of the simplest and yet most profound interventions for helping reduce cardiovascular risk and cardiovascular events."

Renowned cardiologist Stephen Sinatra, MD had this to say about the benefits of earthing: "Reduction in inflammation as a result of earthing has been documented with infrared medical imaging and with measurements of blood chemistry and white blood cell counts."

The Native Americans had it right all along. There's healing power right beneath your feet. If you can't get outdoors and put your bare feet on the earth as often as you would like, there are products that can help to keep you grounded. For instance, I wear an earthing band on my wrist. For more information on earthing products, see the Resources beginning on page 165.

MEDITATING

There are thousands of studies showing that meditation can positively impact mental and physical health by reducing stress, improving sleep, and increasing focus. On a physical level, meditation lowers high blood pressure and levels of blood lactate, which helps reduce anxiety attacks. It also increases serotonin production, and improves the immune system. Meditation relaxes the entire brain, including its emotional center. And there are plenty of ways to meditate. For example, you could simply sit or lie quietly, let your mind go blank and focus on your breathing. Or you could repeat a single word or mantra. Prayer can be a form of meditation. Personally, I believe we're all somehow connected to a Higher Power. I'm also one who thinks that God helps those who help themselves.

I don't do chanting as a form of meditation, but I did try it. I know a number of people who do very well with this form of meditation. As mentioned earlier, I experienced a sort of meditation while chewing my food. The bottom line is that meditation helped open me up to a higher level of understanding—to God, the universal power that controls us all.

EXPLORING ANTHROPOSOPHICAL TREATMENTS

Back when I was working at the Kushi Institute, I went to an anthroposophical doctor who believed in treating the entire body—physical, spiritual, mental, emotional, and social. This type of healthcare encourages people to help themselves and open up to different forms of self-healing. Upon the recommendation of the doctor, I was advised to take mistletoe injections, which have been shown to stimulate the immune system. When you have cancer, you need all the help you can get, so I injected myself with mistletoe in the spleen area for a year. I believed that it was working, especially at the beginning, when I felt flu-like symptoms as my immune system was being stimulated. I felt the injections were right for me. If this is something that interests you, be sure to first consult with your healthcare practitioner to make sure it's the right therapy for you.

UNDERGOING CHEMOTHERAPY

Did chemotherapy work for me? I don't know. All I do know is that it made me sicker than hell. It also made me weak and thin. My body ached like never before, and I had undergone only ten of the eighty prescribed treatments. If I had stuck with all eighty treatments and hadn't walked out of the hospital after only ten, would it have worked? Would I be cancer free? Would I still be alive to tell the story? In my opinion, I probably wouldn't be here today. My body was apparently rejecting the chemo—even the doctor confirmed that. Maybe chemotherapy works for some people. It's up to the individual. Personally, I'm not a big believer in most of it.

TREATING DENTAL ISSUES

In my opinion, amalgam removal is very important in restoring health. Anyone with cancer might want to count the number of silver fillings in his or her mouth. How long have they been there? There is a lot of research to back up how toxic these amalgam fillings can be and what a huge load they place on our immune system.

Dr. Hal Huggins, the father of mercury-free dentistry, spent a big part of his life researching the effects of the mercury poisoning caused by dental amalgams, as well as the dangers of root canals and cavitations (holes in the jawbone where bone or teeth are removed). I personally have seen my blood chemistry results before and after my amalgams were removed, and it was eye-opening. If you're suffering from cancer or any other debilitating disease, I feel that it is a "must" that you see a natural-oriented/biological (holistic) dentist and get his/her opinion. Such a dentist will not only consider your overall health condition, but in most cases will use only biocompatible and non-toxic materials. I'm sure glad I did. See the Resources beginning on page 165 for suggestions on finding a qualified biological dentist.

ELIMINATING HARMFUL MICROORGANISMS

The fact is, we share this world of ours with thousands of harmful creatures both large and microscopically small. It's easy to avoid the ones we can see, but the ones we can't can be a lot more problematic. When it comes to the gut, scientists are discovering that many types of bacteria, both friendly and harmful, reside there. These bacteria can have a direct impact on health. If you have cancer or are suffering from another health condition, you may want to consider the possibility that you might be harboring harmful microorganisms in your gut.

Pesky Parasites

The typical American diet with its processed foods and enormous quantities of sugar, preservatives, and toxic chemicals is nothing but a breeding ground for parasites. Like parasitologist Dr. Bueno told me, he had never seen a case of cancer or AIDS that didn't have a parasitic involvement. He felt it was one of the major underlying causes of disease that too often was overlooked.

Parasites are major suppressors of the immune system. The American Cancer society even admits that certain parasitic worms that are able to live inside the human body can also raise the risk of developing some kinds of cancer. So if you have cancer, it's quite possible that you may also have parasites. One of the first things you should do, in my opinion, is to find out what's bugging you and give them the boot! Parasite test kits and cleanses are readily available. (See the Resources beginning on page 165.)

Yeast

Overgrowth of yeast and fungal infections like *Candida albicans* can compromise the immune system. Scientists studying glucose fermentation in yeast have found that proteins linked to cancer can be activated by glucose (sugar). Some doctors theorize that Candida or other systemic fungal infections can cause or at the very least contribute to the development of cancer. When you examine the link between fungus and cancer further, this makes sense. A systemic Candida infection plays havoc on the immune system. Not only does the immune system become overwhelmed and worn out from fighting the infection, but the fungus excretes toxins that further weaken and harm the body. The major waste product of Candida is acetaldehyde, which produces ethanol, a type of alcohol. Ethanol may be great in cars, but in your body it causes excessive fatigue and reduces strength and stamina. In addition, it destroys the enzymes needed for cell energy and causes the release of free radicals that can damage DNA. Ethanol also inhibits the absorption of iron. Because iron is one of the most important oxygen supports in the blood, ethanol in your body creates low oxygen levels. Deal with Candida if you want to beat cancer.

Fungi

Chemotherapy and radiation cause many changes in the body as they destroy cancer cells. One major change is that they weaken the immune system, which can increase the chances of getting an infection, including a fungal infection. As far back as the 1950s, medical students at Johns Hopkins Medical School were trained to think "fungus" every time solid tumor cancer was discovered in a patient. In fact, they were encouraged to think "fungus" as the possible cause of virtually any serious illness. That's because one of their textbooks, *Fungous Diseases of Man* by J. Walter Wilson, MD, taught them to do so.

Doug Kaufmann of the cable television show Know the Cause has been leading the charge in helping get the word out about how important it is to know the true cause of illnesses. He writes, "More and more practitioners are beginning to see the fungus link to their patients' symptoms and are using dietary changes, prescription and non-prescription antifungals, and other strategies with great success. Maybe the most important thing we could do is minimize those small but frequent exposure points of fungus, mycotoxins, or foods (sugar), and drugs (for example, antibiotics) that exacerbate fungal overgrowth." Doug developed the Kaufmann Diet and Antifungal Program which could prove to be very helpful to anyone who suspects fungus might be an issue.

STAYING POSITIVE

A positive mindset is vital when you're battling cancer. I just can't say this enough. Once you choose a course of action/treatment, it's important to believe 100 percent in what you're doing. Negative people can influence you and make it harder for you to succeed, so don't let anyone undermine your confidence and determination. If there ever was a time in your life when you need every advantage you can get, it's when you're fighting cancer.

For me, a hard-ass attitude worked great. I determined that nothing and no one was going to get in my way and I refused to be defeated. I also refused to cut corners on the healing regimens I adopted. I made up my mind to fight to the end and that's what I've done. It's also important to realize that once you're out of danger, you have to stick with healthy habits. Don't wander too far off the trail of good health care habits or you'll find yourself in trouble again.

HEALING WITH MUSIC

A growing body of research attests that music therapy is more than a nice perk. It can improve medical outcomes and quality of life in a variety of ways. Just as listening to heavy rock metal can raise your heart rate, listening to soothing music can also produce direct biological changes, such as reducing blood pressure and cortisol levels. Upbeat lyrics can increase your level of optimism, too. Music therapy has been found to be effective in:

- **Easing anxiety and discomfort during procedures.** In controlled clinical trials of people having colonoscopies, cardiac angiography, or knee surgery, those who listened to music before their procedure had less anxiety and less need for sedatives. People who listened to music in the operating room reported less discomfort during their procedure. And those who heard music in the recovery room used less opioid medication for pain.

- **Reducing side effects of cancer therapy.** Listening to music reduces anxiety associated with chemotherapy and radiation. It can also help to stop nausea and vomiting for patients receiving chemotherapy.

- **Aiding pain relief.** Music therapy has been tested in a variety of patients, ranging from those with intense short-term pain to those with chronic pain from arthritis. Overall, music therapy decreases pain perception, reduces the amount of pain medication needed, helps relieve depression in patients with pain, and gives them a sense of better control over their pain.

I would often listen to relaxing music for its therapeutic effects and sense of well-being. Music was very healing for me, and I think that any technique you can employ to help you in your battle against cancer is a good thing. I always played music in my room, my car, anywhere I could. Music makes you happier, and happier is healthier!

GETTING QUALITY SLEEP

It's no secret that sleep is vitally important for good health. Without regular, good-quality sleep, it's much harder to heal. I personally believe it's necessary to get eight hours of sleep every night, although I know many people claim they can get by on less. Our bodies regenerate primarily at night when we sleep. In fact, there are certain times of night when different organs are rebuilding.

Are you like many people who find that they fall asleep easily, but wake at the same time in the middle of the night? This can be incredibly frustrating, especially if you can't fall back asleep and wake up tired the next day. The concept of an "Organ Clock" in Chinese medicine can help explain why this occurs. In Chinese medicine, chi (energy) moves through the body's meridians and organs in a twenty-four-hour cycle. Every two hours the chi is strongest within a particular organ and its functions within the body. The body, mind, and emotions are inseparable in Chinese medicine. This means that disharmony in your physical body is tied to your emotional state. So if you wake up at 3:00 AM, when liver energy peaks, you may be suffering from Liver Chi stagnation. This could be related to an unhealthy diet, excess alcohol consumption, unresolved anger, or high levels of stress. If you consistently wake at 4:00 AM, it could be due to a lung imbalance, which is related to grief and sadness, fatigue, or reduced immune function.

I've been pretty lucky when it comes to sleeping. I've always been able to sleep well whether I'm outdoors in a pup tent or indoors on a cotton futon. I'm very grateful for that!

UNDERGOING SURGERY

When it comes to treatment options for any illness or health condition, surgery is anyone's last choice. In some cases, however, it may be necessary. In fact, surgery and a good surgeon might be considered among our best friends during certain circumstances. I've learned that surgery for cancer works best on solid tumors that are contained in one area. It is a local treatment, meaning that it treats only the part of your body with the cancer. In my opinion, surgery can sometimes cause the cancer to spread. That's why I think vitamin C and other healing modalities should be started immediately (and especially after having surgery) to help stop the cancer from spreading and to give your body a healing advantage. Of course, your doctor or healthcare practitioner will recommend the best surgical procedures for your particular needs.

CONCLUSION

This chapter gives an overview of the main ways I fought to outsmart stage IV melanoma. Would I absolutely guarantee they would also cure someone else's cancer? I would not, but really that's not the point. The point is that it was what I did on my journey back to health and it worked for me. It also allowed me the opportunity to learn more about why cancer exists in the first place and what more we can do to fight our own individual battles. Knowing all that I know now, if I were to be diagnosed with cancer today, and based on the things I've learned over the years, I might do things a little differently. In the next chapter, we'll get down to the nitty gritty of my personal list of do's and don'ts when dealing with cancer.

1 1

If I Had It to Do
All Over Again

*"If you don't know where you are going,
you might end up somewhere else."*
—Yogi Berra

Beating cancer was by far the hardest fight I ever fought. I'll never forget lying in the hospital bed, feeling as though I had been thrown in the ring with the heavyweight champion of the world and I didn't even know how to box. Somehow, some way, I had to figure out how to survive. I was grasping for help anywhere I could find it. Thankfully, my prayer was answered. I gained valuable information from the books I read and the people I met along my journey. With sheer grit and determination, I succeeded in taking all I learned and used it to completely change my lifestyle. I not only survived stage IV melanoma, but I'm happy to say that I'm thriving more than thirty years later!

The truth is that there is still no magic bullet for killing cancer. You can ignore, beg, plead, stomp your feet, or whatever . . . but ultimately, you have to roll up your sleeves and go to work if you want to fight this sneaky enemy and win. Cancer is complicated. While there is more than one pathway back to health, navigating the maze of information can be downright confusing. Where do you start? What do you do first? Which diet is best? What is the best way to detoxify? Over the years, I've discovered what I think is most important. In this chapter, I'd like to share with you what I've learned in the hope that it might make your journey a lot easier. No matter what you choose to do, in my opinion and from my personal experience, there are some things that are non-negotiable. Here's what I'd do if I had it to do all over again.

KNOW WHAT QUESTIONS TO ASK

Despite the fact that statistically nearly 40 percent of men and women will be diagnosed with cancer at some point during their lifetime, we don't want to think that we might be one of them. When people are first told they have cancer, they feel as though their world has come to an end— believe me, I've been there! And while your doctor may pause briefly while you catch your breath, and then continue to tell you more about what type of cancer you have and what the next steps will be in treating it, for most, it's not an easy speech to follow—let alone comprehend and ask the appropriate questions. This is all too common and is usually the time when a patient hands over complete control over what happens next.

If this has happened to you, you should make an immediate follow-up appointment. And it's probably best to take along a loved one or invite someone you trust to go with you to help ask questions and even take notes. Write down your questions in advance and take the list with you so that you don't forget anything. And while the answers to some of the following suggested questions may be hard to hear, they are vital to your understanding of what you're dealing with and what you need to do next:

- What type of cancer is it?

- Is it in a single area or has it spread to other parts of the body? Where?

- Is it aggressive?

- What are my treatment options and what would they entail?

- What are the side effects, both short- and long-term?

- What are my odds of recovery? Of being cured? Of it recurring?

- Will my insurance cover the costs of the doctors, drugs, treatment(s) and the hospital stays? Or will I need to pay a portion of it out-of-pocket?

By having these answers to weigh and consider, you will be in a better position to make more informed decisions moving forward.

Know What Your Medical Insurance Covers

Getting well shouldn't be about money, but let's be real. Treatments can be costly. Typically, conventional treatments (for the most part) are covered by health insurance, possibly with deductible and some out-of-pocket expenses. As noted in AARP's "The High Cost of Cancer Treatment," average costs for treatment run in the $150,000 range. Eleven of the twelve cancer drugs that the Food and Drug Administration approved in 2012 were priced at more than $100,000 per year. One study noted that "new, unproven experimental cancer therapy agents can cost more than $60,000 a month for treatment."

If you have Medicare as your primary insurance provider, you need to make sure the doctors and hospitals you work with accept Medicare. While most hospitals do, a number of doctors do not. In addition, you may have a secondary medical insurance provider. Check with them to see what costs they will be able to pick up.

If you decide to treat your cancer using alternative natural healthcare, the costs vary widely depending upon what type of treatment you choose. Check with your insurance provider to see if they do cover such treatments. Unfortunately, most health insurance plans don't cover alternative cancer medical expenses at all. And a lot of people just can't afford to pay for alternative treatments out-of-pocket. If this is you, then you're going to have to do it yourself if you want to survive. But whatever you do, don't throw in the towel! Know that there are many things you can do for yourself to help detoxify and strengthen your immune system. I did it, and you can, too. For example, you still have to eat, so if all you do is change your diet and lifestyle and make changes to optimize your home environment, you'll be surprised how much of a difference it can make. Add just one supplement (maybe some high dose vitamin C) and gain even more benefits! And so on . . . depending upon your budget. We will be covering a number of these things in more detail later in the chapter.

Get A Second Opinion

Mistakes happen. They can be made in labs. Files can be accidentally switched. MRIs can be misinterpreted. Whatever the reason, facts don't lie. Medical errors are now listed as the third leading cause of deaths in America after heart disease and cancer. And although it may seem unfathomable, patients may even be purposely misdiagnosed. It is heartbreaking to read about instances in which unsuspecting patients received inappropriate, even unnecessary, chemotherapy and radiation treatments and even unnecessary surgery.

To those who were either perfectly healthy or whose condition did not warrant chemotherapy, the healthcare fraud they endured is often as devastating as any cancer diagnosis. An example is the case of an oncologist in Michigan who was convicted of submitting $34 million in fraudulent charges to Medicare and private health insurance companies over a period of six years. He pleaded guilty to charges of health care fraud, conspiring to pay and receive kickbacks, and money laundering. Fortunately, he's behind bars now. I can't imagine how outraged I would be if I had been one of his unsuspecting "patients" and tortured with chemotherapy unnecessarily.

If I were newly diagnosed with cancer today, because of my confidence in the natural approach to treating cancer, I would seek the best integrative, functional medicine doctor available in my area . . . or I'd travel as far as I needed in order to find the right one. Such a practitioner is going to be more open to—and familiar with—natural cancer treatments. I'd follow it up with a second opinion—or even a third. If surgery were necessary, which it is in some cases, then I would find the very best surgeon available. Interestingly, according to a poll at McGill Cancer Centre, in a poll of sixty-four oncologists, fifty-eight indicated that they would not utilize chemotherapy for themselves or their families, stating that this form of treatment is "too toxic."

Go Bearing Records

Before you go see another doctor for a second opinion, always be sure to have a copy of your medical records and tests to provide for the new physician, just in case they were not forwarded by your first doctor's staff. Unfortunately, this omission is a common occurrence and only winds up having you reschedule your appointment to a later date—and the last thing you need is to waste valuable time waiting for another appointment. A three-ring binder with your medical history is a great thing to carry along with you . . . just in case. Of course, in some cases, you may need to show the doctor the results of previous MRI or CAT scans. Ask the doctor who requested the tests to be taken for a copy on a CD or flash drive that you can take along. While this may sound like a lot of unnecessary work, I can assure you, it is worth the effort.

Be forewarned that you can't trust someone just because he or she is a natural healthcare practitioner. Do your research. Find out what their track record is. You'll have a better idea if the treatment method is going to work after a short period of time—usually after about three months. Regardless of what care you choose, realize that no one is going to care about you the way you care about yourself. You're going to have both bad and good days, but don't beat yourself up if you get off track—just don't make a habit of it. Tomorrow is a new day.

WEIGH YOUR OPTIONS
AND MAKE A PLAN—IMMEDIATELY

Once you have all the facts, you need to determine your course of action, make a plan, and act fast. Take charge of your own health—if you can. Don't wait for someone else to do it for you. And don't sit in fear hoping cancer will go away on its own. Believe me, I know that's easy to say when you're reeling from a cancer diagnosis—but action, in itself, can be very therapeutic. As I said before, you have no time to lose. There are many things that can be done at home—with or without a doctor's care. They may seem common sense (and they truly are), but don't underestimate them.

We have more control over our health than we may realize. The science of epigenetics is proving what we've always intuitively known—our environment greatly influences our genes. The air we breathe, the foods we eat, the water we drink (or don't drink), how much we sleep, how we handle stress, whether we exercise, and all the other lifestyle choices we make day to day—all can either turn our genes *on* or turn them *off*. Not everyone with the genetic mutations known to cause cancer actually gets cancer. Genes—good or bad—don't switch on and express themselves unless the environment they're in is conducive for this to happen. Put simply, genes may load the gun, but they don't necessarily pull the trigger.

It felt like a sucker punch when I discovered I had a part in creating my cancer. But once I understood that, I realized I had the power to un-create it, too. Our habits, the toxins we're exposed to, the food that we eat, and how we handle our stress—all of these things factor into the disease development process when the body has more than it can handle.

So now the rubber meets the road. You must decide what you're going to do. How badly do you want to live? That may seem like an odd question, but you'd be surprised how many people are willing to give up without a fight—many times just because they think they don't have enough insurance or money. What are you willing to do to change? What *can* you change? If you decide to give it all you've got, then you'll need to use not only your body, but your mind and spirit to win the battle. While there are some cancer risks out there that are beyond our control, many may be just one lifestyle choice away! Why not explore and employ all the options that are at your disposal?

GIVE IT ALL YOU'VE GOT—USING BODY, MIND, AND SPIRIT

We humans are complex beings. We can treat our body as a machine, but if we ignore the emotional and spiritual components of our lives, we may be missing key elements of healing. It's important to address the body as a whole.

You Only Have One Body—Better Take Care of It!

Our bodies make up to a million cancer cells every day, depending on diet and lifestyle. As long as our immune system is functioning properly, these cancer cells are destroyed, and healthy cells flourish. But if our immune system isn't functioning properly, then we're in trouble. A compromised immune system either won't recognize those cells as cancerous or won't have the strength to destroy them. And when the cancer cells multiply upwards to a billion in number, they will start forming tumors.

What do you do? Give your body what it's crying out for! Cancer is your body's urgent call for help—a screaming S.O.S. Now is the time to roll up your sleeves and fight like your life depends upon it . . . because it does. You'll be surprised at some of the simple substitutions you can make in your everyday life that will strengthen, support, and nourish your body—turning it into a true lean, mean, fighting machine!

When you're at war with cancer, you first must quit ingesting toxins. Your focus should be on getting the poisons that are dragging you down out of your body as soon as you possibly can. Load your body, instead, with cancer-fighting foods, probiotics, and supplements so that it will have a fighting chance.

Mind Over Matter

I believe that at least 50 percent of winning the fight against cancer is believing in what you are doing. If you don't have your mind in the right place, then it's going to be that much harder. Through the ups and downs of daily life, you'll need to keep focused on your goal and try to stay as positive as you can. Remember that thinking "I can't do it" will never get you anywhere. Once you've made your plan of action, you simply can't afford to let self-doubt creep in. Take heart—once you begin seeing results, you'll know you're on the right track. After all, seeing is believing, and it helps you to be even more determined to stick with your plan.

The truth is that no one on this earth can escape emotional trauma. In my case, the emotional trauma I suffered as a child due to the untimely deaths of my mother, father, step-brother, and the death of my beloved grandparents was more than I could handle. We can choose to sweep our troubles under the rug, but when traumas are left unresolved, they may cause physical damage to our bodies. How? Our bodies respond to stress with a cascade of hormones and chemicals. We can feel the adrenaline coursing through our veins, often during a moment of fear. We recognize this as the "fight or flight" syndrome. In general, our body returns to homeostasis—a state of balance—in about an hour. But long term or repeated stress continues the release of chemicals even when they aren't needed, resulting in lower immune function and an open pathway for disease.

The Sympathetic Nervous System (SNS) is the primary system involved in this process. If the SNS is stuck in the "on" position, adrenaline and noradrenaline-stimulating mechanisms within it will alter genetic code. This genetic alteration can lead to a number of pro-cancer processes.

Douglas Brodie, MD, a pioneer in understanding the connection between the emotions, the mind, and cancer, noticed after almost three decades of research that the majority of individuals diagnosed with cancer have similar psychological traits. He calls this the "Cancer Personality Profile." Among these characteristics is the experiencing of a traumatizing and emotionally-damaging event roughly two years before getting a cancer diagnosis. The tendency to internalize intense emotions, difficulty in establishing closeness with others, and an inability to adequately cope with stressful situations are other characteristics of the Cancer Personality Profile.

Keep Your Spirit Up

While we can't change the past, we can begin today to find ways to heal the wounds of emotional trauma and reduce chronic stress. Prayer, meditation, and visualization are very helpful. They can be done in the quiet of your home, during your lunch hour at work, or even on the road (day or night). Focus on the positive, be grateful for what you have, and visualize what you want. These suggestions may sound trite, but they are surprisingly powerful. Just like negative thoughts release certain hormones and chemicals in our bodies, positive emotions, such as joy, love, and gratitude also release substances, such as dopamine and oxytocin, two very powerful mood boosters. Go ahead, give yourself a dopamine boost! If you ever needed it, now is the time.

Exercising, taking a walk in the woods, getting out in nature—these are all excellent stress relievers. There is, after all, a direct link between regular exercise and the regulation of stress hormones. Make it a point to get outside and walk every day if you can.

Optimize your vitamin D levels by exposing your skin to at least twenty minutes of sunlight every day. You typically need enough sun exposure to turn your skin a light shade of pink, which means you will produce about 20,000 units of vitamin D. Longer exposures will not produce any additional vitamin D.

Negative self-talk is self-induced sabotage, so avoid it at all cost. Why have enemies when you can beat yourself up perfectly well? Stop and think about the loop you play in your head day and night. Notice anything? If it's full of self-destructive thoughts, then you're defeated before you even start. Instead, learn to rewrite the script that plays in your head. When you catch yourself reverting back to old, familiar negative trains of thought . . . stop! Change the "tape" to include positive messages to yourself.

Misery loves company, but that's no company to keep while you're in the middle of the battle of your life. It's important to surround yourself with positive, like-minded people. It sure made a difference in my life. If you can't find a friend to confide in, consider finding a support group. Make peace with your past for the sake of your health. If you have cancer, if you're under a lot of pressure or negativity from family or friends, if you want to pursue a natural cancer-fighting protocol and you're financially able, then you might consider taking some time to think—maybe even go away for awhile like I did. After all, it's your life you're dealing with. Isn't your life worth doing whatever it takes?

THINGS THAT PROMOTE CANCER

Before I developed cancer, I had no idea there could be so many risk factors. But now I know that there are many everyday substances, exposures, and situations that can lead to cancer (and other diseases). While they may take years to do their damage, the accumulated exposure to these toxins can eventually take a serious toll on our health. The three things absolutely necessary for survival are air, water, and food. You'll want to take great care to ensure all are the best quality possible. By understanding which things promote cancer and what you can do to prevent or help fight cancer, you'll have a much better chance to avoid being just another sad statistic.

ENVIRONMENTAL EXPOSURE

According to the National Institutes of Health, an estimated two-thirds of all cancers are caused by environmental risk factors. While we can't control everything in our shared environment, by being aware of the dangers, we can take steps to eliminate those factors under our control and limit our exposure to others. These include: polluted air, deadly mold, cigarette smoke, radon, EMF radiation, pesticides, and other hazards.

■ Polluted Air

The average person can go (roughly) about three weeks without food, three days without water, but only three minutes without air. While we may not have as much control over the quality of the air we breathe outdoors, there are many precautions we can take to ensure the quality of air we breathe in our immediate indoor environment is healthy.

Polluted Outdoor Air

Some of the common sources of outdoor air pollution include the gasoline vapor and solvents, automobile exhaust, power plant and nuclear plant emissions, acid rain, mold spores, chemicals released from paper mills and smelters, and dangerous chemicals and glyphosates found in pesticides and herbicides (weed killers). Visible sources of air pollution include smoke and particulates from fires, dust, and even the ever-increasing number of chemtrails high in the sky with who-knows-what kind of emissions.

Take precautions when at all possible to limit your exposure to outdoor air contaminants. When pumping gas, stand away from the pump and try not to breathe in the gasoline fumes. If at all possible, avoid living near a nuclear power plant. And don't expose yourself to dangerous herbicides.

Polluted Indoor Air

When we think of air pollution, we tend to think of the quality of air in big, industrial cities. We may not realize it, but the indoor air quality in our homes and work places can be much more polluted than outdoor air. In fact, "Sick Building Syndrome" is an increasingly serious problem as we strive to make our homes and offices airtight. Since our very lives depend on air and our health on good air quality, it is wise to take precautions that the air inside your home is contributing to your health, not harming it.

After you've identified and treated the causes behind any indoor air pollution in your immediate environment, consider putting a good air purifier in place. Air purifiers can help protect you and your family from toxic, harmful contaminants in the air you breathe indoors. Be advised, however, that buying the wrong air purifier may not reduce the most serious contaminants in your indoor air environment to safe breathing levels. The one I use and recommend is the *HealthWay* system. It effectively addresses all three pollutant categories and has been proven to capture 99.99 percent of all particles as small as .002 micron in size. It also eliminates most gases and odors and kills 94 to 100 percent of harmful viruses, molds, and bacteria. For information about recommendations for indoor air filtration systems, see the Resources on page 165 of this book.

In addition, plants are natural air purifiers and are especially good at removing toxins. Aloe Vera helps to rid the air of formaldehyde, bamboo banishes benzene and trichloroethylene, chrysanthemums rid the air of ammonia, dwarf date palms remove zylene (a chemical found in solvents, paints, and adhesives), dracaena (corn plants) help eliminate cigarette smoke, spider plants eat carbon monoxide, and the red emerald philodendron helps remove all indoor toxins. When I was going through my cancer, I made sure to have a lot of these plants in my house.

■ Deadly Mold

Mold in your home, school, or workplace can be a serious concern for your health, since up to 40 percent of American schools and 25 percent of homes have mold infestations. Mycotoxins, produced by some molds, can cross into your brain from your nose and eyes. Two of the better-known toxic molds include *Stachybotrys chartarum* ("black mold"), which can cause everything from headaches to cancer, and *Aspergillus,* which can cause severe lung infections, or progress to whole-body infections. If you suspect mold growing in your home—and especially if you have cancer—you'll want to call in the big guns, the professionals. The visible portion may just be the tip of the iceberg, and the experts know what they're doing. Don't take an unnecessary chance.

■ Cigarette Smoke

Smoking is the leading cause of preventable death in the U.S. At least 69 of the 250 known harmful chemicals in tobacco smoke are known to cause cancer. Do yourself (and everyone around you) a favor and quit smoking. Secondhand smoke is dangerous as well. According to the National Cancer Institute, exposure to secondhand smoke irritates the airways and has immediate harmful effects on a person's heart and blood vessels.

■ Radon

Radon, a radioactive, colorless, odorless gas, is the second leading cause of lung cancer. Radon gas can accumulate in buildings, especially in confined areas, such as basements or even attics. Symptoms from radon poisoning include a persistent cough, wheezing, frequent infections, such as bronchitis or pneumonia, loss of appetite, and more. The only way to know if you are being exposed to high levels of radon in your home is to perform a radon test. You buy these test kits from home improvement stores, hardware stores, or even online. You can also contact the National Radon Defense to find professionals in your area who can help you with continuous radon monitoring and radon mitigation. A radon mitigation system uses ventilation to reduce radon gas concentrations in the air inside your home. See the Resources on page 165 for additional information.

■ EMF Radiation

We love the convenience of cell phones, Wi-Fi, and even crib monitors that add convenience to our life. But the invisible, ever-increasing radiation and electromagnetic exposure from these modern inventions come with a steep price to our health. If you're trying to fight or prevent cancer, be smart and limit your exposure to them.

Every single electron, cell, tissue, and organ in our bodies carries a specific frequency or range. The frequencies emitted by these modern-day conveniences can cause destructive disruptions in our bodies. These disruptions may take years to express themselves as illnesses, but it's a slippery slope and one you'll want to carefully traverse when you are battling cancer.

Avoid talking for more than a few short minutes on your cell phone and use the speaker option when you do. Avoid carrying your cell phone in your pocket or otherwise next to your body. Always turn it on airplane mode or OFF when not in use. Never ever sleep with your cell phone near your body. I installed an old-fashioned landline for my home and save the cell phone for emergencies when I'm away from home.

There are simple measures you can take to shield your router or smart meter—see the Resources on page 165. "You may not be able to see electropollution, but your body responds to it as though it were a cloud of toxic chemicals." —Ann Louise Gittleman author of *Zapped: Why Your Cell Phone Shouldn't Be Your Alarm Clock and 1,268 Ways to Outsmart the Hazards of Electronic Pollution.*

Cordless phones may seem innocent, but they are more dangerous than cell phones. The transmitter base of a cordless phone blasts out high levels of radiation, even when the phone isn't being charged or in use. Radiation from a cordless phone can be as high as 6.5 volts per meter, which is twice as strong as that found within 100 meters of a cell tower. Also avoid baby monitors, or at least place them several feet away from baby's crib.

When you snooze, are you losing out on valuable, health restorative sleep? Then take a closer look at your bedroom. Are you sleeping near an electrical breaker panel? Is it just on the other side of your bedroom wall?

One solution is to move the head of your bed to the farthest wall from the electrical panel. Distance matters! It's the inverse-square law, which simply means that as you double your distance from a source of radiation, you quarter your exposure to it. If moving further away from the electrical panel is out of the question, another solution is to shield the panel by painting your wall with EMF blocking paint. You can measure how much radiation your electrical panel is emitting by using an EMF meter.

Is your head positioned near an electrical outlet while you're sleeping? While an electrical outlet doesn't emit nearly the amount of EMF radiation that an electrical panel can (especially if nothing is plugged in and drawing power from it) your body is still subjected to a small amount of radiation.

So how can you clean it up? Ideally, you could cut off the circuit breaker to your bedroom during the night. If that is not an option, you can unplug all of the electronic devices in your bedroom. Remember, the idea is to get eight hours of restorative sleep, not to bathe our bodies in electromagnetic pollution while we sleep. Turn your bedroom into a healing haven.

■ Pesticides

According to the Environmental Protection Agency, dangerous contaminants (including pesticides) are as much as five times more prevalent indoors as outdoors. That means you could have more residual toxins inside your house than you do in your yard! Children are considered to be more sensitive to chemicals in the environment than the general population due to their size relative to exposure. And when you think about those pesticides sprayed by your friendly local pest control representative along the interior baseboards and the cabinets in your home . . . where your children often crawl and explore . . . it's downright scary. And don't think because the pesticides are "odorless" that they're any less dangerous. Our nose used to warn us to the commonsense danger, but not anymore.

Opt for natural pest control strategies instead. Keep floors and counters as clean and disinfected as possible so as not to attract pests. Essential oils, diatomaceous earth, and other natural solutions are much safer options. For example, consider peppermint essential oil to repel ants, flies, and spiders. Cedarwood is known to help repel roaches, moths, and weevils.

■ Other Hazards

According to the Journal of Occupational and Environmental Medicine, paint exposure may increase cancer risk. "Researchers examining data from the Swedish Cancer Registry and the Swedish census found a 'significantly increased' risk of lung cancer among painters and lacquerers; bladder cancer among artists; and pancreas cancer, lung cancer and non-lymphocytic leukemia among paint and varnish plant workers. Cancer risks for women were elevated for cancers of the esophagus, larynx and oral cavity among lacquerers and for oral cancer among glazers."

Formaldehyde is a known carcinogen, found not only in mortuaries and hair salons, but in plywood and particle board products commonly used in the construction of modern-day furniture. Styrene, used in boats, bathtubs, and in disposable foam plastic plates and cups, may also cause cancer.

As reported by the National Resources Defense Council, scientists from George Washington University, Silent Spring Institute, Harvard University, and the University of California studied common house dust and discovered that homes all across America are chock-full of hazardous chemicals including phthalates, flame retardants, and other toxic chemicals. Phthalates are used in numerous plastic and vinyl materials, cleaning products, and personal care products. Flame retardants are chemicals found in building insulation, electronics, and furniture. These products all shed phthalates and flame retardants into dust.

TOXIC HOUSEHOLD PRODUCTS

Could your choice of cookware or air freshener be harmful to your health? Yes! It's important to know what your household products are made of, and how they might be harming you. Repeated exposures to toxins and chemicals have a cumulative effect. Your body's detoxification systems can only handle so much before they are bogged down and unable to do their job. When these toxins accumulate, illness isn't far behind, including cancer.

■ Household Cleaners

Many household cleaners are more dangerous than the germs they claim to kill. Triclosan, a commonly used antibacterial that is used in everything from hand soaps to toys, has been linked to serious health issues, including thyroid, hormone, and skin problems, simply by being absorbed through the skin. Once studies showed this chemical didn't provide any more antibacterial protection than washing with regular soap and water, public pressure started forcing it out of many products. It is still lurking in many soaps and other personal hygiene products, however, and should be avoided. Also, avoid scented laundry products of all types. Studies show that scented detergents and dryer sheets may contain more than 25 air pollutants, including the carcinogens acetaldehyde and benzene. Benzene causes leukemia and other blood cancers, according to the American Cancer Society. Acetaldehyde has been shown to cause nasal and throat cancer in animal studies.

There are many safe, natural cleaning products available on the market today. Or you can replace toxic household cleaners with inexpensive, natural cleaning solutions. Not only will you save money, you'll be doing your body a big favor. For example, you can use white vinegar in a spray bottle for disinfecting cutting boards, countertops, doorknobs, cleaning windows, and cutting scum in the bathroom shower. Over-the-counter hydrogen peroxide in a spray bottle is another great method of disinfecting countertops and cutting boards. Use baking soda and a brush to scour kitchen sinks. Grind up a lemon rind in the garbage disposal to eliminate odors. Wool dryer balls can be used to eliminate static cling in place of synthetic-fragranced dryer sheets.

■ Dangerous Cookware

I ditched the aluminum and Teflon cookware when I discovered both are harmful to your health. As Dr. Parcells once said, "I'd rather have the most deadly serpent in the kitchen than a single aluminum pot or pan." I don't cook with cast iron either, unless it is Le Creuset cookware. Le Creuset's cookware is made with cast iron, but is finished with a matte enamel, so they don't leach iron. Other good options are clay, ceramic, glass, or heavy gauge stainless steel cookware and bakeware. High-grade stainless steel pots and pans, such as *Saladmaster*, are very good options. Some stainless steel cookware isn't high enough quality and can leach out heavy metals, such as chromium, nickel, and copper. The more nickel the cookware contains, the worse it is for you. Although some of these options are more expensive, don't be foolish and scrimp on something as important as your everyday pots and pans.

CONTAMINATED WATER

All fifty states have water systems that violate the Environmental Protection Agency's Safe Drinking Water Act, so you'll want to avoid drinking unfiltered water from the tap as it can contain toxic chemicals, parasites, and even pharmaceuticals. If you have well water, take care to have your water tested regularly. Avoid drinking from plastic water bottles as they can leach unwanted chemicals, including bisphenol (BPA), an estrogen-like chemical, and antimony, a potential carcinogen.

TOXIC FOODS

Most of us live busy and stressful lives and it's easier just to grab something quick and worry about nutrition later. But real, quality food is vital for good health. If you already have cancer, it's important that you don't fuel the fire by making toxic foods part of your diet.

■ Processed Foods

Avoid processed foods that contain additives, such as MSG, trans fats (partially hydrogenated oils), chemical preservatives, and artificial sweeteners and artificial colors. Avoid non-organic fruits and vegetables—there are upwards of fifty-four pesticide residues on non-organic strawberries and forty-seven pesticide residues on non-organic apples!

You're kidding yourself if you think that the FDA is protecting us from an onslaught of deadly contaminants in our foods. It's up to us as individuals or parents to protect ourselves and our families. I urge you to check out Dr. Renee Dufault's book, *Unsafe at Any Meal: What the FDA Does Not Want You to Know About the Foods You Eat*. Dr. Dufault, former investigator at the FDA, heroically quit her job after being told she couldn't post her eye-opening findings on inorganic mercury and high fructose corn syrup in our national food supply.

Dr. Dufault, along with a team of researchers, analyzed thirteen years of data and conducted a clinical trial to see if processed food intake resulted in higher levels of inorganic mercury (a deadly toxin). They found that simply eating processed foods contributes to higher inorganic blood mercury levels—making you more prone to diseases, such as Alzheimer's, autism, cancer, diabetes, heart disease, and more.

Dr. Dufault: "Most of the public has no idea that the food they eat may contain these substances because of loopholes in the laws, misleading food product labels, and faulty risk assessment processes . . . .when the quality of food has the power to determine how our genes behave and whether or not we will succumb to disease or disability, we cannot ignore the contaminant problems that render much of our food supply unsafe to eat. As a society, we cannot afford to continue to live in an environment where our people are unsafe at any meal."

■ Sugar

Cancer thrives on sugar, so waste no time kicking sugar to the curb! Eliminating this sweet, but deadly, poison from your body is an absolute must. Even fruit must be restricted. Some people recommend fruit in a cancer diet, but I think that if you eat any fruit at all, you'll want to limit it to very small amounts. I didn't eat fruit for over four years, and I survived! But if you opt for eating fruit, you'll want to choose those with cancer-fighting phytonutrients, such as (organic) blueberries, blackberries, raspberries, or strawberries. They are also relatively low in sugar content.

"Cancer feeds on sugars of all kinds—fruit sugar, as well as the glucose that the body makes from grains and other starchy foods. Some people with cancer mistakenly believe that they should only avoid table sugar, but other types of sugar, even the natural sugar that is found in fruit, should be avoided as well." Avoid sugar in all its forms: white sugar, glucose, fructose, sucrose, maltose, lactose, raw sugar, brown sugar, powdered sugar, molasses, maple sugar, honey, corn syrup, high-fructose corn syrup, synthetic sugars, such as sorbitol, mannitol, and xylitol, Nutrasweet, Equal, and alcohol. After a few weeks of eliminating sugar from your diet, your taste buds will begin to "re-set" and you'll gradually become free of sugar cravings. Instead, let the sweetness of vegetables amaze you. Roasting or sautéing vegetables helps to bring out their sweetness.

Satisfy your need for something sweet by enjoying carrots and squashes, such as buttercup, butternut, kabocha, acorn, delicata, and hubbard. Squash contains high levels of beta-carotenes with built-in anti-cancer benefits. Use them in a variety of ways from baking to pureed soups. Delicious and nutritious! Adding a little cardamom, cinnamon, nutmeg, ginger, vanilla, or cloves (in small amounts) can also enhance their flavor. Beware of overdoing it with high amounts of juices, such as carrot juice, because of the overabundance of sugar. Keep juices to a very limited amount.

■ Grains

I love grains, but if I were doing it all over again, I wouldn't be excessive with my grain intake. If you eat grains, eat only the whole grains. And be aware that even those can be loaded with mycotoxins, fungi, yeast, and heavy metals, such as arsenic, cadmium, and lead. Many people are gluten intolerant and have problems digesting glutenous grains. Although they are rich in fiber and can act as a probiotic, many grains are also mucus-producing, so for all these reasons eat them in moderation.

Whatever you do, avoid refined milled or cracked cereal grains and leave the bread on the shelf. If you decide to eat grains, choose grains, such as amaranth, barley, buckwheat, millet, quinoa, polenta or grits, or Basmati rice. These have less arsenic, a dangerous toxin, according to Consumer Reports. In addition, you'll want to avoid most flours except for the occasional almond or coconut flour.

■ Dairy

I highly recommend avoiding dairy. I found that when I ditched the dairy in my diet, not only did my allergies become a thing of the past, but my overall health improved. Mucus-producing foods can clog up your lymphatic system. If cancer cells are trapped in the lymphatic fluid, then it's easier for them to multiply and more difficult for your hardworking white blood cells to access them and destroy them.

I do, on occasion, enjoy small amounts of grass-fed, organic butter or ghee (clarified butter). I actually prefer organic ghee, which is rich in beneficial nutrients and contains several fatty acids that are important to health. It has a higher smoking point than butter, so may be used in cooking. I also like *Follow Your Heart* cheeses (made from coconut oil) that are usually available in your health food store.

■ Risks of Eating Out

In my opinion, if you have cancer, it's better not to eat out. The quality of water, food, and food preparation are, at best, unpredictable. I know this because I travel quite a bit, and it isn't always easy to find restaurants with healthy selections. There are times, of course, when eating out is unavoidable. Your best option will often be a restaurant that serves organic, locally grown or farm-to-table foods. Don't be afraid to ask for what you need or for your special dietary requirements. Most of these types of restaurants will try to be sensitive to your needs. I feel so strongly about this that I made this a focus of my Wellness Foundation. See the Resources on page 165 for more information.

THINGS THAT HELP PREVENT AND/OR FIGHT CANCER

Make your body a fortress! Turn on your body's natural immune fighting defense systems! There are many things you can do beginning this very day to give your body what it needs to fend off disease and to repair itself, beginning with the basics.

CLEAN, PURE WATER

Clean, pure, properly filtered water should be a top priority. Water is vital in nourishing every cell in your body and removing waste and toxins. Get yourself a good water filter for your home. All water filtration systems are not created equal, and what you may need for your home in Houston is not what will work in New York City. There are different contaminants in each water supply, and you need specific filters to address it. You need to at least have a filter at your tap for your drinking and bathing water—the water you use for showering and bathing is absorbed into your skin. Consider a shower or bathtub filter for the bathroom and an over-the-counter or an under-the-counter filter for the kitchen. Even better (if you can afford it) is to opt for a whole-house water filtration system.

Personally, I'm not a fan of reverse osmosis systems as they remove much needed minerals from water. I prefer a combination ceramic and carbon filtration system. The one I use and recommend removes 99 percent of parasites, bacteria, dirt, rust, sediment, chlorine and other chemicals, 99 percent of glyphosate and herbicides, 98 percent of heavy metals, including lead, aluminum, iron, mercury, nickel and zinc, 95 percent of pharmaceutical compounds, and 92 percent of fluoride. A good system should filter down to 0.5 microns for particles. See the Resources on page 165 for more information on recommended water filtration and water testing.

Exposure to Bisphenol A (BPA) in plastics has been linked to cancer. As a substitute for plastic water bottles, I prefer bottling my own water to take with me in a glass or stainless-steel container.

CANCER-FIGHTING FOODS

When I was on the macrobiotic diet, I ate almost all of these cancer-fighting foods on a daily basis. No wonder the diet works! It's not a coincidence that most of these foods were recommended—it makes sense. In my opinion, the more of these foods that you can ingest, the better off you'll be. Food can indeed be thy medicine!

Always choose organic, non-GMO foods when possible. They're worth the extra cents they cost. Besides avoiding dangerous pesticides and fungicides which non-organic produce may contain, organic produce contains significantly more vitamins and nutrients. An organic apple has 300 percent more vitamin C than a non-organic apple. Shop at farmers' markets or grow your own. When you can't avoid non-organic produce, be sure to wash and peel fruits and vegetables before eating. We're trying to rid our bodies of toxins, not take on more.

There are many diets out there but, unfortunately, there's not a "one size fits all". What works for one person may not work for another. If you're not prescribed a diet, there are some basic things to keep in mind that are, in my opinion, non-negotiable. First of all, take note of the powerful cancer-fighting foods. Make a list if you need to and keep it in your pocket or purse when shopping. If you have cancer or are trying to prevent cancer, you'll want to load up on cancer-fighting foods.

Cruciferous vegetables*, in particular, are powerful foods that help to detox heavy metals and synthetic estrogens out of the body. Be sure to include them in your daily diet. The powerful and cancer-fighting foods listed in Table 11.1 are best when they are organic.

POWERFUL FOODS THAT WORK FOR YOU			
HERBS, BEANS AND BEAN PRODUCTS, AND VEGETABLES			
Arugula*	Black-Eyed Peas	Burdock Root	Carrots and carrot tops
Asparagus	Bok Choy*	Cabbage* (red and green)	Cauliflower*
Avocado	Broccoli*		
Adzuki Beans	Brussels Sprouts*		

HERBS, BEANS AND BEAN PRODUCTS, AND VEGETABLES (CONTINUED)

Celery and Celery Root	Green Peas	Mushrooms (Bella, Cremini, Reishi, Shiitake)	Rutabaga*
Chickpeas	Horseradish*		Scallions
Chives	Jerusalem Artichokes	Mustard Greens*	Sea Vegetables
Cilantro (helps with heavy metal toxicity)	Kale*	Natto (fermented soy beans)	Snap Beans
	Kidney Beans	Navy Beans	Split Peas
Collard Greens*	Kohlrabi*	Onions	Sprouts (broccoli, garbanzo, lentils, mung)
Cucumber	Land Cress*	Parsley	
Daikon Radishes*	Leeks	Parsnips	Squash (particularly buttercup and kabocha)
Dandelion root and greens	Lemon Juice	Peppers (red, green, or yellow)	
Endive	Lentils	Pinto Beans	Turnips* (roots and greens)
Escarole	Lettuce—Romaine, Iceberg	Pomegranate	Wasabi*
Garden Cress*	Lotus Root	Pumpkin	Watercress*
Garlic	Mung Beans	Radish*	Zucchini
Green Beans			

NUTS AND SEEDS

Almonds (raw)	Cilium Husks	Macadamia Nuts	Sesame Seeds (white or black)
Apricot Pits	Flaxseed	Pumpkin Seeds (raw or lightly roasted)	Sunflower Seeds
Chia Seeds	Hemp Seeds		Walnuts

HEALTHY OILS

Avocado	Flaxseed	Olive (cold-pressed, unfiltered extra virgin)	Sesame
Coconut (organic, virgin, cold-pressed and unrefined)	Hemp		Walnut
	Macadamia	Pine Nut	

BEVERAGES

Coffee*	Green Tea	Mugwort Tea (helps combat parasites)	Water (pure, clean, filtered or spring water)
Dandelion Root Tea	Kukicha Twig Tea (be sure it is certified radiation-free)	Pau d'arco Tea (made from the inner bark of the tree)	
Essiac Tea			
Graviola Tea			

*My favorite is pesticide-free Purity brand coffee, which has over 60 percent more antioxidants than other organic brands, and is lab tested to certify it is free of mold, mycotoxins, and pesticides. See the Resources on page 165.

■ Seaweeds

Seaweeds contain compounds that can inhibit cancer cell growth and prevent metastasis. Kombu and arame (brown seaweeds), dulse (a red seaweed), kelp, wakame, and nori are common options. Avoid hijiki as it is consistently shown to possess high levels of heavy metals, particularly arsenic. Be sure to source your seaweed products from non-contaminated waters, such as the southeastern coast of Argentina or the Patagonian shores. Ideally, obtain them from a company that tests their products for contamination. Check out the Resources on page 165 for recommendations for safe seaweeds.

■ Herbs

There is a wealth of healing herbs available—many are as effective as pharmaceuticals and much safer. You'll want to get familiar with nature's medicine cabinet! Cilantro, arugula, garlic, and onions are amazing (and tasty) natural chelators of heavy metals in your body. Burdock is a member of the daisy family—its roots contain health-promoting antioxidants, including quercetin, luteolin, and phenolic acids and is used to combat cancer and improve arthritis. Oregano is an herb that can reduce inflammation, fight bacterial, fungal, viral and parasitic infections, and even shrink tumors. Thyme is a member of the mint family and can lower blood pressure and cholesterol levels and is a cancer fighter.

■ Spices

I discovered some powerful spices that I put to work for me on a daily basis. For example, instead of regular "table salt," I opted for Celtic sea salt. It is rich in eighty-four minerals and trace elements. I don't recommend using black pepper if you have cancer. Black pepper contains safrole (banned by the FDA after it was found that injecting large amounts caused liver cancer in lab rats). Instead, I would opt for cayenne pepper. Cayenne has anti-fungal properties and is a circulatory stimulant for our digestive and lymphatic systems.

Turmeric is one of my favorites! It's a golden spice that delivers some powerful benefits due to its high amounts of the antioxidant called curcumin. I also like cinnamon—another of the most beneficial spices on earth.

Curcumin and cinnamon are both known for their anti-inflammatory, anti-oxidant, antimicrobial, immune-boosting, and cancer-fighting properties.

■ Proteins

I believe, in most cases, if you have cancer you should restrict animal protein in your diet since some amino acids that are commonly found in animal protein, especially leucine and tyrosine, can stimulate cancer growth. In addition, the enzymes that your pancreas produces (trypsin and chymotrypsin), which are the important enzymes for digesting proteins—and even more important in the destruction of cancer cells—are used up faster by eating too much meat. Your enzyme bank suffers. We want to give our body all the fighting tools it needs to defeat cancer. There are certain people, however, that may benefit from small, moderate amounts of animal protein.

From what I have studied and read, people with lymphomas, sarcomas, myelomas, and melanomas may have a certain metabolic type that requires more protein. If you choose animal proteins, it's best to avoid or limit red meat and select, instead, small amounts of white meat chicken or turkey. You can also enjoy wild-caught white meat fish, such as cod, flounder, haddock, halibut, snapper, sole, and (occasionally) trout. Salmon, shrimp, and lobster may also be enjoyed occasionally. Limit seafood to two to three times per week because it has been found to have relatively high mercury levels. (Mercury is one of the most toxic, immune-suppressive substances on the planet and has long been connected to a host of health issues, including cancer.)

Boiled or poached pasture-raised, organic eggs are acceptable proteins. Once your cancer is under control, you can consider increasing animal proteins gradually. Of course, beans and bean products such as those listed on our recommended food list, (see page 140), may be enjoyed as a protein on a regular basis.

■ Probiotics

Probiotics are vital to good gut health and can lower your cancer risk by helping your immune system operate at peak performance. We must have a strong immune system, and the gut flora represents up to 80 percent of our immune system. I also eat organic, unpasteurized miso soup on a regular basis, and moderate amounts of sauerkraut (*Bubbies* is my favorite brand). Also beneficial are unpasteurized organic pickled vegetables and kimchi (a side dish made from salted and fermented vegetables), natto (a traditional Japanese dish consisting of fermented soybeans) and occasionally tempe—all of which help to boost the level of healthy gut flora . . . and ultimately, our immunity.

SUPPLEMENTS

When you're fighting cancer, you need all the help you can get to optimize your immune system. Along with a healthy diet and lifestyle, quality supplements can have a tremendous effect on your health and give you the boost you need to combat cancer. You wouldn't go to war with only one soldier and a small amount of ammo. Likewise, in the war against cancer, it's important to arm yourself with as many key helpers as possible.

As mentioned in Chapter 8 (The Vitamin C Connection), I believe high dose vitamin C therapy is one of the key things you can do for your health, especially as our bodies don't produce vitamin C and must be supplemented. At the very least you'll want to be sure you're taking a good quality multi-vitamin and other supplements that contain antioxidant, anti-inflammatory and anti-cancer properties. Antioxidants such as Astaxanthin (550 times stronger than vitamin E and 6,000 times more potent than vitamin C), Resveratrol, Quercetin, Berberine and Curcumin are also excellent choices.

Additionally, thymus, spleen, and bone marrow supplements are great ways to support your immune system. White blood cells are key disease fighters and are produced in the bone marrow, thymus and spleen. Supporting these immune producing heroes makes sense. Thymus stimulates the development of T cells. The spleen plays multiple supporting roles, acting as a filter for blood and helping to fight infection. Blood marrow is the primary source of lymphocytes. All of these help promote immunity. Note: Glandulars should be from New Zealand or Argentina where animals are raised hormone-free and are carefully tested and monitored.

I also believe that enzymes are one of your greatest defense mechanisms against cancer. As far back as 1906, Dr. John Beard, a Scottish embryologist, proposed that pancreatic proteolytic digestive enzymes represent the body's main defense against cancer. Dr. William Donald

Kelley and, later, Dr. Nicholas Gonzales took up the good fight and successfully treated many cancer patients (particularly those with pancreatic cancer) using enzyme therapy.

Enzymes not only decrease inflammation, they increase the defense power of macrophages, powerful white blood cells. They work by digesting the fibrinogen layer (membrane) that cancer cells and tumors have, thereby enabling the immune system to recognize that it needs to attack! Enzymes also help break down and assimilate nutrients and minerals in the body and assist with digestion. It's interesting to note that if you have cancer, there's a good chance your reserve enzymes are low. Consult with your healthcare practitioner or someone familiar with enzyme therapy to determine how much works best for you.

Although not a prerequisite for everyone, here are the core supplements I take on a daily basis as a preventative measure. Regardless of whether you are treating or preventing cancer, you must find the best quality supplements available—this is no time to skimp on quality. Please consult with your health care practitioner for the right program for you. See the Resources on page 163 for recommended brands.

CORE SUPPLEMENTS	
SUPPLEMENT	**DOSAGE**
Astaxanthin	12 mg 1x daily with meals
Berberine	500 mg 2 to 3x daily
Bone Marrow (grass-fed from New Zealand)	500 mg 3x daily with meals
Co-Q 10	200 mg 2x daily with meals
Colon Cleanser	As directed on label
Cracked Cell Chlorella (mercury-free)	2,000 mg 2x daily
Curcumin	500 mg 3x daily with meals
EGCG Green Tea Extract	1,500 mg 2x daily with meals
Fish Oils (high in EPA and DHA and molecularly distilled)	1,000 mg 3x daily with meals
Lysine	3,000 mg 2x daily with meals

SUPPLEMENT	DOSAGE
Magnesium	400 mg 1 to 2x daily with meals
Methylated B Complex	As directed on label
Multiple Vitamin	As directed on label
Organic Apricot Pits (high in vitamin B-17) (A soft large seed similar to an almond)	3 pits 1 to 2x daily as a snack
Organic Powdered Greens	As directed on label
Pancreatic Enzymes	As directed on label
Probiotics—Acidophilus, Bifidus and L. Plantarum, plus inulin, a special prebiotic substance (dairy-free, gluten-free, soy free)	30 to 40 billion beneficial bacteria 2x daily on an empty stomach
Proline	3,000 mg 2x daily with meals
Quercetin	1,000 mg daily
Raw Thymus (Glandular—bovine)	500 mg 3x daily with meals
Raw Spleen (Glandular—bovine)	1,000 mg 3x daily with meals
Resveratrol	500 mg 2x daily
Vitamin A	25,000 IU 1 to 3x daily with meals
Vitamin C (tablet or liquid form)	10,000 to 16,000 mg spread throughout the day (with meals)
Vitamin D-3	2,000 IU 1 to 2x daily with meals
Vitamin E	400 IU 1 to 2x daily with meals

DETOXIFICATION

Detoxing is serious business when you're dealing with cancer. The chronically ill person's body is like a big city with garbage collectors on strike. You have to open the detox drains and get the poisons out—the sooner the better. If you're eating a lot of vegetables and fiber and drinking a lot of pure water, you should be able to eliminate after each meal—or at least twice a day. If not, it's a sign that you may need a little help.

■ Coffee Enemas

Coffee enemas are a great help for removing toxins. Dr. Nicholas Gonzalez advised cancer patients to administer enemas up to twice a day, but once or twice a week might be fine for some. You'll want to check with your doctor or health care practitioner to find out what is best for you. When coffee is introduced to the colon, it is absorbed into the bloodstream and carried to the liver, where it helps to increase the production of glutathione, sometimes known as "the mother of all antioxidants". Glutathione is used by every cell in the human body. And of course, use organic, pesticide free coffee and unbleached coffee filters. If you're skittish about enemas, consider colonics, also known as colonic irrigation or colon hydrotherapy. It should be done by a qualified practitioner.

■ Far-Infrared Saunas

In an article in the *Townsend Letter for Doctors and Patients*, Lawrence Wilson, MD, wrote, "If I were to single out one method to combat cancer, it is the sauna. It assists removal of chemical toxins and heavy metals, increases oxygenation, enhances the immune system, and reduces the radiation burden in the body." Infrared sauna treatments are harmful only to malignant cells that just can't take the heat! Normal, healthy cells are immune to infrared radiation. Other ways of eliminating toxins from the body include daily exercise, sweating, dry brushing, yoga, and deep breathing. These are available on the market and can be done in your own home. See the Resources on page 165 for recommendations.

■ Oxygen Therapies

Oxygen therapies can be effective ways of killing cancer cells. Healthy cells love oxygen, but cancer cells do not. When oxygen is administered at high pressure rates, up to twenty times more oxygen can be absorbed by the bloodstream. This oxygen is transported to damaged organs and tissue, which speeds up both healing and recovery time. Consult with your healthcare practitioner to determine what is right for you.

There are several things you can do at home, as well, to oxygenate your body. Exercise, hiking, plain old-fashioned walking, and deep breathing can all be very beneficial. You can reap all the benefits in about thirty minutes a day! If you are a runner or an exercise extremist, go easy because it's best that you don't stress your body while you're in the healing stage. Gyms are fine but think about it—you're breathing everyone else's toxins. To me, it makes more sense to go outside to exercise or exercise in a clean air space at home.

Hyperbaric Oxygen Therapy (HBOT)

Used for over fifty years to repair burns and heal chronic wounds, increased systemic oxygen works by stimulating the immune system and the overall healing process. One way that HBOT affects cancer cells, is by reducing hypoxia, a low-oxygen condition that is common in cancerous tumors.

Ozone Therapy

Ozone therapy is well-respected in many parts of the world, but is not widely accepted in the U.S., though in my opinion it should be. In Germany, for example, ozone therapy is the standard of care used by 70 to 80 percent of practicing physicians. When you consider that ozone takes a mere ten seconds to kill 99 percent of bacteria, fungi, yeast, mold, and viruses—3,500 times faster than chlorine—it's easy to see why it's so effective. It has even been shown to kill cancer cells upon contact.

Hydrogen Peroxide Therapy

Hydrogen Peroxide Therapy works by stimulating natural killer cells, which attack cancer cells. When hydrogen peroxide is taken into the body (orally or intravenously) it increases the oxygen content of the blood and body tissues dramatically. Oxidative therapies also increase the production of interferon, which is required to combat infections as well as cancer.

Caution: *The hydrogen peroxide sold over the counter at your local pharmacy (3 percent hydrogen peroxide) should NEVER be ingested orally. Only food grade hydrogen peroxide (35 percent) is recommended for internal use and must be properly diluted down to 3 percent with water. Consult with your healthcare practitioner.*

■ Healthy Body Products

We often think of our skin—the largest organ of our body—as a detoxification route, and certainly our bodies can do that through sweating.

However, it's a two-way street. Our skin also absorbs whatever we put on it. And isn't it odd that we accept the fact that medicine can be transmitted via transdermal patches, while we don't even consider the onslaught of unwanted chemicals that we put on our skin every day through our use of common body care products?

Avoid body care products, shampoos, and deodorants with chemicals, such as DEA (used as a foaming agent in shampoos), parabens, and BHT (used as a solvent in many nail polishes and lipsticks). Lipsticks can contain lead, and mascara can contain mercury—heavy metals you definitely don't want in your body. Avoid shampoos, perfume, and lotions that are heavily scented, as they contain phthalates, a hormone disruptor. Instead, use natural body care products and cosmetics that are chemical-free. Look for products with the fewest ingredients or make your own! Coconut oil, for example, is a simple, one-ingredient body lotion that actually nourishes your skin. Baking soda makes a simple, inexpensive deodorant. I like and use *Weleda* products.

If you're concerned about the body products you're using or considering using, visit the Environmental Working Group's *Skin Deep* website where they have a database of products. You will find the contact information for these and other references in the Resources on page 165.

■ Dental Issues

Your oral health directly impacts your overall health. Now is the time to take note of any dental issues you may have. Neglect your teeth and gums, and it's not only your mouth that will suffer. According to the National Institutes of Health, "There are many studies indicating that cancer patients are manifested with poor oral health." Do you have a lot of amalgam fillings? They are very hazardous to your health—50 percent of the amalgam is mercury, one of the most poisonous substances on the planet. How about root canals? According to the Toxic Element Research Foundation (TERF): " . . . it is no coincidence that in the U.S. root canals have been found to abound in people with Multiple Sclerosis, Lou Gehrig's disease, Lupus, leukemia, diabetes, arthritis, and a host of other autoimmune diseases.

Reversal of these diseases, as shown by improvements in physical conditions as well as positive changes in blood chemistries, occurs after the removal of dental toxic challenges (mercury, nickel, aluminum, root canals and cavitations) in conjunction with stimulation to the immune systems of these people." If your dental health isn't up to par, you'll want to find a good naturally-oriented (biological) dentist to help you remove and replace amalgam fillings and even root canals safely and to assist you in restoring and maintaining good oral health. See the Resources on page 165 for recommendations.

■ Synthetic Fibers

Man-made fabrics such as acrylic, nylon, polyester, and rayon are treated with thousands of harmful toxic chemicals during production. According to a Stockholm University study referenced in *Science Daily*, the highest concentrations of two of the chemicals were found in polyester. Having synthetic fabrics next to your skin, whether wearing them or sleeping with them, just doesn't make sense.

Synthetic Clothing

Many of the clothes manufactured these days are synthetic. For example, most sportswear contains hazardous chemicals, such as phthalates, dimethylformamide (DMF), and perfluorinated chemicals (PFCs). Moisture wicking clothing is supposed to be helpful, but they're synthetic, too. If you have cancer, I suggest avoiding it. Wear natural fabrics instead, such as cotton, linen, or wool.

Synthetic Mattresses and Toppers

Synthetic mattresses often contain petroleum-based chemicals, toxic foams, and fire-retardant chemicals. These chemicals can off-gas even when the mattress is ten years old and there's no chemical smell! Beware of memory foam mattresses and toppers, too. Unless the memory foam mattress is manufactured with organic latex, it is made up of chemicals and man-made substances. I prefer sleeping on an organic cotton futon. These are great because they can be placed directly on the floor, a bed frame, or on top of another mattress—whatever works best for you. For recommended options, see the Resources on page 165.

■ Testing

Even your favorite GPS gadget knows that you can't get to where you're going without knowing where you're starting from. If you don't have cancer (and especially if you do), it is wise to keep an eye on your level of accumulation of known toxins. Testing is the only reliable way. Be aware that routine medical tests often do not reveal our actual risks—some healthcare practitioners are more stringent when interpreting the test results. Also, some typically prescribed blood tests may not even include one of the most important levels you should know: your stored iron, or ferritin level.

The Iron Time Bomb

Do yourself a big favor and have your ferritin level checked. Your ferritin level is an indication of how much iron your body is storing. Too little iron and you're considered anemic. But too much iron is even more common and can be deadly. Even though iron is a required nutrient, people with abnormally high iron levels in their blood are unwittingly creating a perfect environment for cancer cells. I fell into that category—it's surprising how many people do! Routine blood tests typically do not test for the level of iron stores (ferritin level) in your blood, but it's easy to request an inexpensive, simple blood test for this, even without a doctor's prescription (see the Resources on page 165).

The ideal ferritin range is 40 to 50 ng/mL for women and 50 to 60 ng/mL for men. I learned that no matter how much I exercised and watched what I ate, if I didn't prevent my iron from becoming too high, I was overlooking a major element of health. There are no symptoms from excess iron alone. The only "symptoms" are from the disease that excess iron causes—cancer, diabetes, neurological diseases, or a heart attack. It's the silent killer. Fortunately, I discovered ways of reducing the levels of excess iron. In addition to watching my diet, I make sure I donate blood regularly, as each blood donation can reduce the ferritin level an average of 30 to 50 ng/ml.

Nagalase Testing—Cancer Biomarker

Nagalase (short for N-acetyl-galactosaminidase) is a natural enzyme found in the body. High levels of Nagalase in the blood stream are linked to tumor processes. Nagalase is found in cancer cells, which use this enzyme to actively penetrate through connective tissue or collagen in order to metastasize. Increased activity of nagalase has been detected in the blood of patients with a wide variety of cancers, including cancer of the prostate, breast, colon, lung, esophagus, stomach, liver, pancreas, kidney, bladder, testes, uterus and ovary, mesothelioma, melanoma, fibrosarcoma, glioblastoma, neuroblastoma and various leukemias. The Nagalase Blood Test is used to determine the amount of nagalase in your body which can allow early detection of cancer, improving your chances of survival. For more information on this test, please see the Resources on page 165.

Marker Blood Tests

Cancer marker blood tests can be very helpful in determining what your cancer risk is. When cancerous tumors form, they release proteins into the bloodstream, and these can act as markers for cancer. There are many such tests on the market today, and a new one called CancerSEEK. It works by identifying the markers for eight proteins and sixteen gene mutations that are associated with eight common cancers: breast, lung, colorectal, ovarian, liver, stomach, pancreatic, and esophageal.

TREATMENTS AND THERAPIES

It is important to remember that there are many different ways of treating health disorders. Our established medical system is but one way to treat various disorders. As long as you keep an open mind to other modalities and always ask questions, you will be in a better position to make informed decisions. Here are two approaches to treating your health conditions that I have found helpful for myself.

■ Chiropractic Care

We sometimes think of chiropractic care only when our back is out, but regular chiropractic care can be a great asset when fighting cancer. It is beneficial for alleviating pain, reducing stress, and improving mood and sleeping habits. But it does much more than that. Because the immune system interacts directly with the nervous system, chiropractic adjustments can remove obstructions with the signaling pathways between the two systems, directly stimulating the body's immune system.

▪ Professional Healthcare Providers

If you're not a do-it-yourselfer, you might want to consider working with proven alternative health practitioners or successful specialty treatment centers. You'll find some of my recommendations in the Resources on page 165. Before making a decision, call and talk to them. Always learn as much as you can about the people with whom you hope to work.

CONCLUSION

When I began my personal journey of battling cancer, fate stepped in and I was unexpectedly handed the very keys to my healing, which changed the course of my life. Over the years, I have learned so much about what we can do to increase our odds of beating this beast. I truly hope that some of these ideas will prove helpful to you, too. It's much like peeling an onion as you uncover layer after layer of toxins . . . but you have to start somewhere. I realize the list of "things to avoid" and "things to do" can seem overwhelming, but if all you do is to avoid the toxins that are known to cause cancer, you'll have taken a giant first step.

We tend to get so busy just living our lives that we don't take time to care for ourselves the way we should. I fell into that category, and it's part of the reason I found myself in such a dire situation. And when we're young, we think we have all the time in the world, not considering that the bad habits we may be forming will eventually catch up with us. The good news is that we can learn from our mistakes. Once we are aware and awake to the causes of cancer and the part we may have played in its formation, we are faced with the choice of what we're willing to do about it. By focusing on doing all we can to strengthen our body, we'll be in a much better place to fight the onslaught of toxins that bombard us from all directions. Hopefully, the day will come when our society will (purposely and conscientiously) create better solutions to make our shared environment, as well as our food and water supplies, much safer for all of us.

In the last chapter, I'd like to share with you where I am today, where my journey led me. Was it all worth it? Including the cancer diagnosis? I'd honestly have to say that although it was a very difficult and painful road, it was worth it all. Hindsight is indeed 20/20. The end result is that I am living my best life NOW, and I am excited to pass along all I've learned to anyone seeking help (and hope) in their battle against cancer.

12

Putting It All Together

"If you are going through hell, keep going."
—WINSTON CHURCHILL

Through my journey, I learned there is one very powerful antidote to the fear that grips you when you hear the words, "you have cancer"—and that is knowledge. When I was first diagnosed with stage IV melanoma, I felt like it had sneaked up on me out of nowhere. Certainly, everything changed in an instant when I heard those three dreaded words. It seemed like my life was over at the age of thirty-two when I felt like I was just getting started and things were finally going my way. I didn't realize that I had a part in creating the cancer that had suddenly become my personal Public Enemy #1. I thought I was doing all the right things while keeping my eyes focused on sidestepping heart disease. Turns out I was wrong about that, too.

One thing that cancer will teach you is how to get your priorities straight. My list of what was truly important got really short, really quick. I had to take a long hard look at what I was doing to take care of myself. It forced me to set aside my pride. My motivation to find a way to stay alive suddenly took center stage. I prayed what probably was the first genuine prayer of my life—it was certainly one of the most heartfelt—and I was shocked when it was answered so thoroughly and so fast. You may not get three knocks on the door like I did, but now that I've discovered the keys to good health, I've dedicated my life to helping others find the same.

The sad fact is that, according to the National Cancer Institute, more than 4,700 new cancer diagnoses are handed down each day. That's well over one and half million Americans who are told they have cancer each year. We need to either be prepared . . . or ready to fight if the time comes

155

that we're one of the unfortunate ones to hear those dreaded words. The treatments I got happened to be the right treatments at the right time. Fortunately, as you've read in the previous chapter, there is a lot more information available these thirty plus years later! The truth is that there are many things people can do to help themselves avoid or overcome cancer. This is the story of how I beat cancer on my own terms, but there are a number of other options as well. As long as you do the work to learn about these options, you can make better, more informed decisions.

My journey has taught me that I have more control over my health than I once thought. Science is proving it. The research of epigenetics suggests that our inherited genes do not necessarily reflect our destiny. Biology alone does not necessarily determine our destiny. We can have an influence over our genetic make-up. We now understand how each of us can be dramatically affected by our environment, diet, stress, and even our thoughts and emotions. The good news is that each of us has the ability to control many of these factors!

Thanks to the teachers and healers I encountered along the way and all the things I learned, I eventually got a better understanding of the toxic overload that caused my body to finally say *enough*. My body had reached its tipping point. Those years of working at gas stations had exposed me to a lot of lead and the dangerous chemical, benzene, at the gas pumps. The carpet installation work I did exposed me to high concentrations of formaldehyde and acetaldehyde. For several years, I was exposed to toxic PVC glues while installing sprinkler systems. The harmful chemicals in the foods I ate was yet another challenge that weakened my body, and the parasites from dealing with my cattle, hogs, dogs and cats, along with numerous trips south of the border also contributed to my toxic overload. Long distance running and working out in the gym while eating a diet low in nutrition didn't help me out at all. And added to all of that, the trauma and emotional stress I experienced throughout my early life only contributed to my problem.

It's absolutely astounding that we are being exposed to an estimated 85,000 chemicals on the market today. This extraordinary quantity of chemicals has had a history of so few controls that they are now permeating every corner of our increasingly contaminated environment. Even chemicals that studies prove are known cancer-causing agents may very well be in our homes and offices. It is up to us to choose wisely. Our body's detoxification systems, though wonderfully made, can handle only so much before they are bogged down and unable to eliminate all the poisons we come in contact with. When these toxins accumulate, illness isn't far behind—and that can include cancer.

I learned that I had to reduce my toxic overload if I wanted to pull out of the mess I was in. According to Dr. William Lee Cowden, MD, board-certified cardiologist, clinical nutritionist, internist, and cancer expert, the key to recovery from cancer and autoimmune disease is to strengthen the resistance of the host. Strengthening resistance means getting your immune system in good fighting shape. That entails getting toxins out of the body, which may be impairing your body's resistance and adding in nourishing lifestyle practices to optimize your immune system. I learned that I could reduce my toxic overload by being aware of (1) what I put *into* my body; (2) what I put *onto* my body; and (3) the environment I chose to be in. I learned, too, that I had to either handle my emotional stress or it would handle me. Our everyday choices can work either for us or against us. We may not be able to reduce 100 percent of the stressors, but we can do a lot. By reducing toxic burdens to the body and providing the quality nutrition it needs, it is amazing what the body can do to repair itself.

At first, I didn't realize that I had the power to reverse a lot of the damage which had already been done. But as I made small but important changes, my body responded favorably. I could feel the difference. My energy increased, my appetite improved, and little by little, day by day, my body healed itself. Some cancers may grow undetected for a decade or more. Knowing that, you can choose to do something now or simply hope for the best. Just like it took time to push my body to the brink of disaster, the small lifetime shifts I made significantly changed my health . . . for the better. I learned that my body is self-healing when I stopped bombarding it with poisons, gave it what it needed, and got back as close to nature as possible. Now I know that cancer does not need to be a death sentence. It was, instead, my body's loud and clear wake-up call—a wake-up call I totally respect today.

If I had to sum it all up, I'd say that the key to overcoming cancer is to gain knowledge—that needs to be your first focus. You must take control of your health and do your research. Weigh your treatment options. If you need to go off somewhere by yourself to think about your choice of treatment or what you're up against, go to the mountains, a place of worship, or someplace that is near and dear to your heart—do it, but don't dally around. Remember that there are people out there who will take advantage of you, so always learn as much as you can about the people who you hope to work with.

It is vitally important to point out that there is more than one pathway to overcoming your cancer. Whether you choose the do-it-yourself method or work with a health practitioner or a cancer clinic, remember that there are things you can begin doing today that will help to fortify your body to defend itself. No matter which path you choose, roll up your sleeves and prepare to go to battle. You are in charge. Start by getting rid of the poisons in your body any way you can. Begin feeding your body healthy, quality cancer-fighting food and good probiotics. Like Dr. Parcells once said, if you want to live to be 100, there are certain things you have to do. If we don't wake up and start taking care of ourselves, we might not make it to age 100. Stay active and keep your mind busy. Find your purpose. Life can be wonderful when you feel good about yourself, take care of yourself, laugh and tell jokes, spend time with your loved ones, and do whatever it is that you enjoy. Surround yourself with people who feel the same way. And once you've done all that, stay steady at the helm and keep going! Watch what your body can do when you treat it right.

Maybe even more importantly, through my journey I found my true calling. After I recovered from cancer, the last thing I wanted to do was to squander my second chance at life. I didn't want to go back to selling beer and cigarettes at convenience stores as I had done before. Instead, after waking up at two o'clock one morning with the name "Uni Key: universal key to health" in a dream, I knew what I wanted to do. I created Uni Key Health Systems, Inc. For many years, I consulted with clients one-on-one, and by observing different patterns, I developed the Uni Key line of products. I'm happy to say that Uni Key has been tremendously successful in helping thousands of people find their keys to good health. For nearly thirty years, my mission has been to motivate and inspire others to take charge of their health—no matter how big or small their challenges may be.

Coming face to face with death and making the long journey back to health made me respect the fact that good health is one of God's greatest gifts and should never be taken for granted. Not only did I gain a deeper, personal understanding of the dreaded disease called cancer and how to fight it, but it changed me on many levels. And although I wouldn't wish it on anyone, I know that the experience made me a better person. My battle with cancer taught me many lessons that I probably wouldn't have learned any other way . . . and gave me the bonus of a new purpose in life.

Life is precious. We're all here for a reason. We can help each other by sharing what we've learned. My wish is that you will enjoy a long, healthy, and happy life . . . and that if you are battling cancer, you, too, will someday be able to share your success story with others and say, "I used to have cancer . . . but I don't anymore!"

EPILOGUE

My Life Today

*"It's your road . . . and yours alone. Others may walk
it with you, but no one can walk it for you."*
—Rumi

I'm blessed beyond measure today. What seemed like the end of the
world over thirty years ago turned out to be an amazing journey with
twists and turns I never could have imagined. As I crisscrossed the country, I met and was inspired by some of the most fascinating teachers I've
ever known. I've been privileged to share the past twenty-eight years of
my life with one of them —Ann Louise Gittleman, an extraordinary, tireless health warrior and award-winning author.

I now reside in the beautiful State of Idaho where Uni Key Health Systems, Inc., is headquartered. I travel frequently to my other location in
Houston. From its humble beginning in a small room in the back of my
house, Uni Key has grown over the past twenty-seven years to a robust
company with a team of dedicated people in all time zones of the continental U.S. I've always insisted upon the most stringent testing procedures for all our products, as I know firsthand how important quality is.
It has not only been my purpose in life, but my greatest honor to help others. If you'd like to check out Uni Key Health, you can find us on the web
at www.unikeyhealth.com.

One of the things that always kept me going was to figure out a way
to stick around and be healthy for my daughter. My dream came true. I'm
happy to say that Carol began working for me after she graduated college. She is now the marketing director for Uni Key Health and works at
the Houston location. It's terrific to have her involved in my business and
my life on a regular basis. Carol is married to Blaise, a wonderful young

man and successful entrepreneur, and I am blessed with a healthy young grandson, Caleb. I enjoy spending time with him every chance I get and watching him grow up.

Though we live many miles apart, my sister, Judy, and I remain close. Through all the years, she remains my steadfast lifeline. It's been such fun spending time over the years with my nephews skiing, boating, fishing, hiking, kayaking, or just sitting around swapping stories. Sometimes we even fire up the ol' Jeep and go for a ride. I continue to love the outdoors and make it a point to practice what I preach by keeping fit. I dare say that I can still keep up with most guys younger than me!

I plan on spending many years to come—as long as I can—continuing to help people and to develop quality products that can get to the root cause of health problems. One of my projects is the Templeton Wellness Foundation. I created the Foundation to give hope to those dealing with a cancer diagnosis or those who are looking for ways to prevent cancer. As a cancer survivor for over thirty years, I've spent a lot of time over those three decades learning how to improve my health. There was no way I could hold back from letting others in on what I had learned from the healers and educators I met on my crazy journey. I know how important it is to roll up your sleeves and get down and dirty with this enemy called cancer. I'm determined to use my second chance at life to give back as much as I can to helping others.

My hope for the Foundation is that it might be a user-friendly comprehensive site to gather information and resources so that no one has to spend countless hours trying to find that needle in a haystack. The Foundation is also interviewing as many people as it can who have had advanced stage cancer like I did and who have survived ten years or more. I want to document and showcase the *living proof* that cancer *can be* defeated. The gift of hope that we survivors can pass on to others is, I believe, vitally important.

Also through the Foundation, we will share recommendations for alternative healthcare practitioners, clinics, promising new products, the latest research, and even healthy restaurants all across the country that you can feel comfortable visiting. I don't usually recommend eating out if you have cancer, but sometimes in a pinch, you aren't given a choice. I didn't have that advantage all those years ago. I cooked for myself while on the road, so I understand why finding restaurants that serve healthy food can be so important. I created an interactive restaurant guide so that you might have healthy restaurant alternatives at the push of a button. I invite you to check it out at www.templetonwellness.com

I am living my best life now. I have traveled all over the world and continue to meet some of the most interesting and informed people on the planet. I enjoy spending time with friends—both old and new. Like the old saying goes, make new friends, but keep the old—one is silver and the other gold. I am rich in friendships!

I don't have to be as strict today with my diet and regimen as when I was in the middle of my fight with cancer, but I *prefer* to stay on track. One of my sayings is to "go out and enjoy life, but always keep one foot on the path to good health!" People call me a born storyteller and I guess I am. I think that's one of the things that is too often missing in this modern day—people used to pass along family lore in the stories they shared from generation to generation. These stories let us know where we came from and reassure us that we have the ability to survive and thrive despite the fact that life is often hard. We can learn from others, without having to repeat the same mistakes.

With age comes an increased desire to give back, to share what we have learned on our journeys. I hope my experience is an encouragement to anyone who hears those three dreaded words, "you have cancer." Look to others who have found a way to beat the odds and defy the statistics. It's what made the difference for me. May you, too, be richly blessed in the path you choose. Let me leave you with these final words, God helps those who help themselves!

Resources

This resource guide is divided into the following sections:

1. **Books**
2. **Diagnostic Tests**
3. **Foods**
4. **Lifestyle Aids**

5. **Medical Professionals & Clinics**
6. **Restaurants**
7. **Supplements**
8. **Websites**

For a complete list of resources, check the Templeton Wellness Foundation website at www.templetonwellness.com

1. BOOKS

Some of these books truly changed my life and served as a guide for my desperate fight back to health. Others I discovered while already well along my journey. All have proved enormously helpful. This is my recommended reading list for anyone dealing with cancer.

Benedict, Dirk. *Confessions of a Kamikaze Cowboy*. Garden City Park, NY: Square One Publishers, 2006.

Cameron, Ewan, and Linus Pauling. *Cancer and Vitamin C*. New York: Warner Books, 1979.

Cowden, W. Lee, and Connie Strasheim. *Create a Toxin-Free Body & Home Starting Today*. Mill Valley, CA: ACIM Press, 2014.

Cowden, W. Lee, and Connie Strasheim. *Foods That Fit a Unique You*. Mill Valley, CA: ACIM Press, 2014.

Dispenza, Joseph. *Healer: The Pioneer Nutritionist and Prophet*. Boyne City, MI: Harbor House, 2012.

Dispenza, Joseph. *Live Better Longer*. Bloomington, IN: iUniverse, 2001.

Gittleman, Ann Louise. *Guess What Came to Dinner?* New York: Avery, 2001.

Dufault, Renee Joy. *Unsafe at Any Meal*. Garden City Park, NY: Square One Publishers, 2017.

Gittleman, Ann Louise. *The New Fat Flush Plan*. New York: McGraw-Hill Education, 2016.

Gittleman, Ann Louise. *Zapped*. San Francisco, CA: HarperOne, 2011.

Kaufmann, Doug A. *The Fungus Link*. Rockwall, TX: Media Trition, 2000.

Ober, Clint, Stephen T. Sinatra, and Martin Zucker. *Earthing*. Laguna Beach, CA: Basic Health Publications, 2010.

Rees, Camilla R. G. *The Wireless Elephant in the Room*. Scotts Valley, CA: CreateSpace Independent Publishing Platform, 2017.

Sattilaro, Anthony J., with Tom Monte. *Living Well Naturally*. Boston, MA: Houghton Mifflin, 1985.

Sattilaro, Anthony J., with Tom Monte. *Recalled by Life*. New York: Avon Books, 1984.

2. DIAGNOSTIC TESTS

In connection with your search for the underlying causes of your health issues, certain diagnostic tests are available as convenient at-home tests, while others can be requested by your healthcare practitioner.

Adrenal Stress Panel
Website: www.unikeyhealth.com/
adrenal-stress-panel
Phone: 800-888-4353

Chemical Toxicity (GPL-TOX: Toxic Non-Metal Chemical Profile)
Website: www.greatplainslaboratory.
com/gpl-tox
Phone: 800-288-0383

DNA Genetic Cancer Risk Profile
Website: https://www.lifeextension.
com/vitamins-supplements/
itemLC100057/DNA-

Expanded GI Panel
Website: www.unikeyhealth.com/
expanded-gi-panel
Phone: 800-888-4353

Genetic Genie (Methylation & Detox Analysis)
Website: http://geneticgenie.org

Nagalase Testing
Website: www.hdri-usa.com

Oncotype DX Breast Recurrence Score
Website: www.oncotypeiq.com

Salivary Hormone Test
Website: www.unikeyhealth.com/
salivary-hormone-test
Phone: 800-888-4353

SpectraCell Laboratories (Telomere Testing)
Website: www.spectracell.com/
patients/patient-telomere-testing
Phone: 800-227-5227

Tissue Mineral Analysis
Website: www.unikeyhealth.com/
tissue-mineral-analysis
Phone: 800-888-4353

23andMe (Genomic Testing—DNA)
Website: www.23andme.com
Phone: 800-239-5230

uBiome (Microbiome Testing)
Website: https://ubiome.com

Your Future Health (Omega Fatty Acids Test)
Website: www.yourfuturehealth.com
Phone: 877–468–6934

3. FOODS

Finding quality, healthy foods is vital for good health. Here are a few of my favorite options.

■ BEVERAGES

Eden Organic Teas
Website: www.edenfoods.com

Organic Oolong Tea
Website: www.arborteas.com/
organic-oolong-tea

Purity Coffee
Website: www.puritycoffee.com
844-787-4892

Roasted Dandelion Root Tea
Website: www.traditionalmedicinals.
com/products/
roasted-dandelion-root

The Tea Crane Oolong Tea
Website: www.the-tea-crane.com/
collections/favorites/oolong-tea

■ BONE BROTHS

Kettle & Fire Bone Broths
Website: www.kettleandfire.com
Phone: 415-857-0024

Pacific Foods Bone Broths
Website: www.pacificfoods.com
Phone: 503-692-9666

■ CONDIMENTS & SWEETENERS

Ginger People Ginger Juice
Website: https://gingerpeople.com

**Health Gems Ancient Five Scalar
Salt**
Website: http://healthgems.com

Nutramedix Stevia Sweet Herb
Website: www.nutramedix.com/
stevia-sweet-herb

Ojio Organic Yacon Syrup
Available on Amazon

Pure Yacon Syrup Gold
Website: http://goldsourcelabs.com/
pure-yacon-syrup

Real Salt
Website: https://realsalt.com
Phone: 800-367-7258

Red Boat Fish Sauce
Website: http://redboatfishsauce.com

**Selina Naturally Celtic Sea Salt
Products**
Website: www.selinanaturally.com

**Swanson PureLo Lo Han Sweetener
(Monk Fruit)**
Available on Amazon and in some
nutritional supplement stores

■ DAIRY & NONDAIRY

**Follow Your Heart Non-Dairy
Cheeses**
Website: https://followyourheart.
com/vegan-cheese

Nancy's Organic Yogurts
Website: http://nancysyogurt.com

■ FISH & SEAFOOD

Best Atlantic Seafood Brands
Website: www.thenourishinggourmet.
com/2014/05/finding-seafood-
untouched-by-fukushima.html

Copper River Seafoods
Website: www.copperriverseafoods.
com
Phone: 888-622-1197

EcoFish
Website: www.ecofish.com
Phone: 603-430-0101

Sustainably Raised or Harvested Low-Mercury Fish Sources
Website: www.nrdc.org/oceans/ seafoodguide

Sustainably Sourced (Farmed or Fished) Seafood
Website: www.cleanfish.com

Wild Salmon Seafood Market
Website: http://wildsalmonseafood. com
Phone: 206-217-3474

■ GRAIN-FREE FLOURS, WRAPS & CRACKERS

Doctor in the Kitchen Flackers
Website: www.drinthekitchen.com

Jilz Gluten Free Crackers
Website: https://jilzglutenfree.com

Organic Gemini Tigernut Flour
Website: https://organicgemini.com

Paleo Wraps from Julian Bakery
Website: https://julianbakery.com

Raw Wraps
Website: www.rawwraps.org

Siete Tortillas
Website: https://sietefoods.com

Simple Mills Sprouted Seed Crackers
Website: www.simplemills.com

■ HIGH-VIBRATIONAL & ORGANIC FOODS

Vervana
Website: www.vervana.com
Phone: 800-228-1507

■ MEATS

ButcherBox
Website: www.butcherbox.com
Phone: 855-981-8568

US Wellness Meats
Website: http://grasslandbeef.com
Phone: 877-383-0051

■ OILS & FATS

Omega Nutrition Hi-Lignan Flax Oil
Website: www.unikeyhealth.com/ products/organic-flax-oil
Phone: 800-888-4353

Plant Proteins
Uni Key Health Fat Flush Body Protein
Website: www.unikeyhealth.com
Phone: 800-888-4353

■ PROBIOTIC & PREBIOTIC FOODS

Bubbies
Website: http://bubbies.com

Eden Ume Plum Vinegar
Website: www.edenfoods.com

Farmhouse Culture Organic Kraut
Website: www.farmhouseculture.com

■ OHSAWA

Available on Amazon and in some nutritional supplement stores.

South River Miso
Website: www.southrivermiso.com
Phone: 413-369-4057

■ SAFE SEAWEEDS

Power Super Foods Seaweed
Website: www.powersuperfoods.com. au/seaweed.html

Watersteps Black Label Gourmet
Organic Roasted Seaweed Snack
Website: www.watersteps.com.au/
products/seaweed

■ SEEDS, NUTS & NUT BUTTERS

Apricot Pits/Seeds
Website: www.apricotpower.com

**Organic Living Superfoods—Life's
Nuts**
Website: http://
organiclivingsuperfoods.com

■ OTHER RESOURCES FOR FINDING HIGH-QUALITY FOODS

American Farmers Network
Website: www.
americanfarmersnetwork.com
Phone: 800-817-6180

American Grassfed
Website: www.americangrassfed.org
Phone: 877-774-7277

**Community Alliance with Family
Farmers**
Facebook: www.facebook.com/
famfarms
Phone: 530-756-8518

**Community Involved in Sustaining
Agriculture**
Website: www.buylocalfood.org
Phone: 413-665-7100

The Cornucopia Institute
Website: www.cornucopia.org

Phone: 608-625-2000

The Eat Well Guide
Website: www.eatwellguide.org
Phone: 212-991-1930

Eat Wild
Website: www.eatwild.com
Phone: 253-759-2318

The Food Routes
Website: http://foodroutes.org
Phone: 814-571-8319

**Garrett Valley Sugar Free Turkey
Bacon**
Website: www.garrettvalley.com

The Grassfed Exchange
Website: www.grassfedexchange.com
Phone: 256-996-3142

The Land Institute
Website: https://landinstitute.org
Phone: 785-823-5376

Local Harvest
Website: www.localharvest.org

**Organic Farming Research
Foundation**
Website: http://ofrf.org
Phone: 831-426-6606

Organic Trade Association
Website: www.ota.com
Phone: 802-275-3800

National Farmers Market Directory
Website: http://nfmd.org

4. LIFESTYLE AIDS

Clean air, pure water, safe cookware, and EMF protection are just some of the
valuable resources you'll want to consider for your home.

■ AIR PURIFIERS

Clean Water Revival (CWR)
Website: www.cwrenviro.com
Phone: 800-444-3563

Cookware & Bakeware
Insta-Pot (Pressure Cooker)
Website: https://instantpot.com

Le Creuset
Website: www.lecreuset.com

Saladmaster
Website: www.saladmaster.com
Electropollution

Aulterra
Website: https://aulterra.com

Earthing
Website: www.earthing.com

The Earthing Institute
Website: www.earthinginstitute.net

EMF Protective Shungite Jewelry &
   Home Goods by Shungite Queen
Website: www.shungitequeen.com

Greenwave
Website: https://greenwavefilters.
   com
Phone: 800-506-6098

LessEMF
Website: www.lessemf.com
Phone: 800-506-6098

■ HOME REMEDIATION

Environmental Relative Moldiness
   Index (ERMI)
Website: www.envirobiomics.com

International Institute for Bau-
   Biology & Ecology
Website: http://hbelc.org

National Radon Safety Board
   (NRSB)
Website: www.nrsb.org

Phone: 866-329-3474

ServPro
Website: www.servpro.com

■ NATURAL & NONTOXIC CARPETING

EarthWeave
Website: www.earthweave.com

Nature's Carpet
Website: www.naturescarpet.com

■ NONTOXIC MATTRESSES

Abundant Earth
Website: www.abundantearth.com

Elemental Green
Website: www.elementalgreen.com

The Futon Shop
Website: www.thefutonshop.com

Naturepedic
Website: www.naturepedic.com

■ PERSONAL CARE & HOUSEHOLD CLEANING PRODUCTS

Aubrey Organics
Website: www.aubrey-organics.com

BeauCle Skin Care
Website: www.unikeyhealth.com/
   beaucle-ultra-hydrating-moisture
Phone: 800-888-4353

Dr. Bronner's Organic Soaps,
   Products
Website: www.drbronner.com

Earth Easy
Website: www.eartheasy.com

EarthWeave
Website: www.earthweave.com

Eminence
Website: www.eminenceorganics.com

EWG Skindeep Cosmetic Database
Website: www.ewg.org/skindeep

Green Shield
Website: www.greenshieldorganic.
com

Melaleuca
Website: www.melaleuca.com

Mrs. Meyer's
Website: www.mrsmeyers.com

Osmosis Skincare
Website: www.osmosisskincare.com
Phone: 877-777-2305

Seventh Generation
Website: www.seventhgeneration.
com

Shaklee
Website: www.shaklee.com

Weleda
Website: www.weleda.com

Zum Zum
Website: www.indigowild.com

■ SAUNAS

Relax Far Infrared Sauna
Website: www.relaxsaunas.com
Phone: 800-533-4372

Sunlighten Saunas
Website: www.sunlighten.com
Phone: 877-292-0020

■ WATER FILTRATION

AIoWater Filters with Metalgon
Website: www.unikeyhealth.com/
under-counter-ultra-ceramic-water-
filter
Phone: 800-888-4353

Aquasana
Website: www.aquasana.com

Berkey Water Filters
Website: www.berkeyfilters.com

Crown Environmental Products
Website: unikeyhealth.com
Phone: 800-888-4353

pH Prescription Water
Website: www.phprescription.com

pHenomenal Water
Website: www.phenomenalwater.com

5. MEDICAL PROFESSIONALS & CLINICS

Finding a good healthcare practitioner that shares your philosophy is vital when you're battling something as serious as cancer. These are a few I highly recommend.

**American Academy of Anti-Aging
Medicine**
Website: www.a4m.com/find-a-
doctor.html

**American Academy of
Environmental Medicine**
Website: www.aaemonline.org
Phone: 316-684-5500

William Lee Cowden, MD
Academy of Comprehensive
Integrative Medicine (ACIM)
Website: www.acimconnect.com
Email: info@acimconnect.com

Institute for Functional Medicine
Website: https://www.ifm.org/
find-a-practitioner

Linda L. Isaacs, M.D. (The Gonzalez Protocol)
Website: www.drlindai.com
Phone: 212-213-3337

The Oasis of Hope's Contreras Alternative Cancer Treatment (C-ACT)
Website: www.oasisofhope.com
Phone: 1-888-500-4675

Naturopathic Physicians
Website: www.naturopathic.org

Paleo Physicians Network
Website: http://paleophysiciansnetwork.com

Re-Find Health
Website: https://re-findhealth.com

Dr. Stephen T. Sinatra, Cardiologist
Website: www.drsinatra.com

■ GERSON (CERTIFIED PRACTITIONERS)

Gerson Practitioners
Website: www.gerson.org

Dr. Miven Donato, GPC, DC, DPT, MT (Medford, Oregon, USA)
Website: http://doctordonato.com

Dr. Vidya Krishnamurthy, GPC, MD (Alpharetta, Georgia, USA)
Website: www.georgiawellnessclinic.com

Dr. Annie Juneau, GPC, ND (Laval, Quebec, Canada)
Website: https://vitacru.com

Nicolae-Ovidiu Lungulescu, GPC, MD (Severin, Romania)
Email: ovidiu7@protonmail.com

Dr. Henry McGrath, GPC, Dip Acu, Dip TCM, ND, MA, MT (Bristol, United Kingdom)
Website: www.henrymcgrath.com

Dr. Melania Nagy, GPC, ND (Budapest, Hungary)
Website: https://gerson.org/gerpress/gerson-health-centre

■ BIOLOGICAL DENTISTS

Consumers for Dental Choice
Website: www.toxicteeth.org/dentistsDoctorsProducts.aspx

Dental Amalgam Mercury Solutions (DAMS)
Website: www.dams.cc

Holistic Dental Association (HAD)
Website: http://holisticdental.org/find-a-holistic-dentist

Huggins Applied Healing
Website: https://hugginsappliedhealing.com

International Academy of Biological Dentistry & Medicine (IABDM)
Website: https://iabdm.org

Dr. Tom McGuire's Mercury-Safe Dentist Directory
Website: www.dentalwellness4u.com/freeservices/find_dentists.html

Talk International
Website: www.dentalwellness4u.com/freeservices/find_dentists.html

■ MACROBIOTIC RESOURCES

Kushi Institute of Europe (Amsterdam, the Netherlands)
Website: www.macrobiotics.nl
Phone: 011 31 20 625 7513
Email: kushi@macrobiotics.nl

George Ohsawa Macrobiotic Foundation
Website: www.ohsawamacrobiotics.com
Phone: 530-566-9765

Planetary Health, Inc.
Websites: www.
macrobioticsummerconference.com,
www.amberwavesofgrain.com,
www.makropedia.com

Phone: 413-623-0012

6. RESTAURANTS

We've scoured the country in search of restaurants that offer real, healthy food options while also adhering to our strict ingredient, preparation, and environmental standards of quality to find you smart choices for eating out without sacrificing your health. To find a recommended restaurant in your area, please see the interactive online map created by Templeton Wellness Foundation.

Templeton Wellness Foundation
Website: www.templetonwellness.com

7. SUPPLEMENTS

Unfortunately, our food supply is lacking in sufficient vitamins and minerals. When you're fighting cancer, you need all the help you can get.

American Biologics Inf-Zyme Forte
Website: www.unikeyhealth.com/
    products/inf-zyme-forte

American Nutraceuticals Vitality C
Website: www.888vitality.com
Phone: 888-848-2548

Nutricology
Website: www.nutricology.com/
    pancreas-pork-720-vegicaps

Phone: 510-263-2000

Dr. Mattias Rath Health Foundation
Website: www.dr-rath-foundation.org

UNI KEY Health Systems, Inc.
Website: www.unikey.com
Phone: 800-888-4353

8. WEBSITES

The following websites contain valuable health information that is regularly updated.

**Ann Louise Gittleman, the First
    Lady of Nutrition**
Website: www.annlouise.com

Doug Kaufmann—Know the Cause
Website: www.knowthecause.com

Templeton Wellness Foundation
Website: www.templetonwellness.
    com

Uni Key Health
Website: www.unikeyhealth.com

References

Chapter 1

"Battle of San Jacinto." History.com. June 12, 2018. www.history.com/topics/battle-of-san-jacinto

Fixx, James F. "The Complete Book of Running." New York: Random House, 1977.

Gross, Jane. "James F. Fixx Dies Jogging." *New York Times*, July 22, 1984. Accessed June 27, 2018. www.nytimes.com/1984/07/22/obituaries/james-f-fixx-dies-jogging-author-on-running-was-52.html

Haas, Robert. "Eat to Win." New York: Signet, 1983.

"Jim Fixx." Wikipedia. June 12, 2018. https://en.wikipedia.org/wiki/Jim_Fixx

Chapter 2

"Hyperthermia to Treat Cancer." American Cancer Society. July 31, 2018. www.cancer.org/treatment/treatments-and-side-effects/treatment-types/hyperthermia.html

Chapter 3

Sattilaro, Anthony J. *Recalled by Life*. New York: Avon Books, 1984.

Sattilaro, Anthony J., with Tom Monte. *Living Well Naturally*. Boston: Houghton Mifflin, 1984.

Chapter 4

Annis, Bonnie. "Cancer's Dirty Little Secret." Cure: Cancer Updates, Research & Education. June 6, 2016. www.curetoday.com/community/bonnie-annis/2016/06/cancers-dirty-little-secret

Rogers, Monica Kass. "Macrobiotic Diet." Web MD. July 6, 2018. www.webmd.com/diet/a-z/macrobiotic-diet

Chapter 5

"Anthroposophy." August 4, 2018. Wikipedia. https://en.wikipedia.org/wiki/Anthroposophy

"George Ohsawa." Wikipedia. July 12, 2018. https://en.wikipedia.org/wiki/George_Ohsawa

"Kukicha." Wikipedia. July 16, 2018. https://en.wikipedia.org/wiki/Kukicha

Kushi, Michio. *The Book of Macrobiotics: The Universal Way of Health, Happiness & Peace* Garden City Park, NY: Square One Publishers, 2012.

"Sagen Ishizukka." Wikipedia. July 12, 2018. https://en.wikipedia.org/wiki/Sagen_Ishizuka

Elwell, Gaella. "Our Story." South River Miso Company. July 12, 2018. www.southrivermiso.com/store/pg/100-Our-Story-History-Full-Text.html

Kienle, Gunver S, et. al. "Anthroposophic Medicine: An Integrative Medical System Originating in Europe." *Global Advances in Health and Medicine* 2, no. 6 (2013). 20–31. doi: 10.7453/gahmj.2012.087

"What Is Macrobiotics?" George Ohsawa Macrobiotic Foundation. July 16, 2018. https://ohsawamacrobiotics.com/gomf-home/what-is-macrobiotics

Yamamoto, Shizuko. *Barefoot Shiatsu: Whole-Body Approach to Health.* New York: Japan Pubns, 1979.

Yamamoto, Shizuko, and Patrick McCarty. *Barefoot Shiatsu: The Japanese Art of Healing the Body Through Massage.* New York: Avery Publishing Group, 1998.

Chapter 6

Gittleman, Ann Louise. *Guess What Came to Dinner?* New York: Avery, 1993.

Scott, Dana. "Pumpkin Seeds: A Natural Solution for Worms." Dogs Naturally. August 13, 2018. www.dogsnaturallymagazine.com/pumpkin-seeds-natural-worms-dogs

Chapter 7

"Chakras and Glands." Chakras.info. August 18, 2018. www.chakras.info/chakras-glands

Dispenza, Joseph. *Healer: The Pioneer Nutritionist & Prophet.* Boyne City, MI: Harbor House, 2012.

Dispenza, Joseph. *Live Better Longer.* Lincoln, NE: Authors Choice Press, 1997.

Chapter 8

Chen, Q., M.G. Espey, et al., "Pharmacological Ascorbic Acid Concentrations Selectively Kill Cancer Cells: Action as a Pro-drug to Deliver Hydrogen Peroxide to Tissues." *Proceedings of the National Academy of Sciences* 102, 38 (2005): 13604–13609. Sep. 6, 2018. www.ncbi.nlm.nih.gov/pubmed/16157892

"Dr. Matthias Rath–Biography." Dr. Rath Health Foundation. April 5, 2017. www.dr-rath-foundation.org/2017/04/dr-matthias-rath-biography

"Heart Disease." Dr. Rath Research Institute. Aug. 30, 2018. www.drrathresearch.org/drrath-discoveries/heart-disease

Klenner, Frederick R. "Observations on the Dose and Administration of Ascorbic Acid When Employed Beyond the Range of A Vitamin In Human Pathology," *Journal of Orthomolecular Medicine* 13, 4th quarter (1988). Sep. 7, 2018. http://orthomolecular.org/library/jom/1998/articles/1998-v13n04-p198.shtml

Levy, Thomas E. "The Clinical Impact of Vitamin C: My Personal Experiences as a Physician." Orthomolecular.org. Sep. 18, 2018. http://orthomolecular.org/resources/omns/v10n14.shtml

Levy, Thomas E. *Curing the Incurable: Vitamin C, Infectious Diseases, and Toxins.* 3rd Edition. Henderson, NV: MedFox Publishing, 2011.

McIntosh, James. "Collagen: What is it and what are its uses?" Medical News Today. June 16, 2017. www.medicalnewstoday.com/articles/262881.php

O'Melveny Woods, John. "Dr. Hal Alan Huggins, Noted Dental Pioneer, Passes Away," *Integrative Medicine: A Clinician's Journal* 14, 1 (2015). Sep. 12, 2018. www.ncbi.nlm.nih.gov/pmc/articles/PMC4566458

Rath, M., and L. Pauling. "Plasmin-Induced Proteolysis and the Role of Apoprotein(a), Lysine, and Synthetic Lysine Analogs." *Journal of Orthomolecular Medicine* 7 (1992). 17–23. August 30, 2018. www.drrathresearch.org/publications/leading-publications/167-plasmin-induced-proteolysis-and-the-role-of-apoprotein-a-lysine-and-synthetic-lysine-analogs

Weir, Hannah K., Robert N. Anderson, et al. "Heart Disease and Cancer Deaths–Trends and Projections in the United States, 1969-2020." *CME Activity* Vol. 13 (November 17, 2016). Sep. 7, 2018. www.cdc.gov/pcd/issues/2016/16_0211.htm

Wright, Jonathan. "Frederick R. Klenner M.D., The Originator of Successful High-Dose Intravenous Vitamin C Therapy." The Alliance for Natural Health USA. July 7, 2018. http://www.anh-usa.org/frederick-r-klenner-m-d-the-originator-of-successful-high-dose-intravenous-vitamin-c-therapy

Chapter 9

Compton, Karen. "For Patch Adams, Good Health is a Laughing Matter." Mother Earth Living. Sep. 11, 2018. www.motherearthliving.com/health-and-wellness/for-patch-adams-good-health-is-a-laughing-matter

Kehoe, John. "The World's Leading Authority on Mind Power." MindPower. Sep. 12, 2018. www.learnmindpower.com/about-john-kehoe

Sinatra, Stephen T. "The Healing Power of Laughter." Heart MD Institute. Oct. 3, 2018. https://heartmdinstitute.com/stress-relief/healing-power-laughter

"Stress Weakens the Immune System." American Psychological Association. Sep. 11, 2018. www.apa.org/research/action/immune.aspx

Sukhoterina, Yelena. "There Is No Cancer There." Alternative Healthworks. Sep. 25, 2018. https//althealthworks.com/16984

Chapter 10

"A. Clinton Ober." ESD Journal. Oct. 4, 2018. www.esdjournal.com/articles/cober/bio.htm

"Candida Infections Cause Some Cancers." Cancer Fighting Strategies. Sep. 19, 2018. www.cancerfightingstrategies.com/fungus-and-cancer.html

Drew, Kyle. "Fungal Infection Mistaken for Cancer?" Doug Kaufmann's Know the Cause. Apr. 10, 2017. www.knowthecause.com/index.php/contributor-blog/46-kyle-drew/4330-are-you-sure-you-have-the-right-diagnosis

"The Health Benefits of Meditation." The Art of Living. Sep. 19, 2018. www.artofliving.org/us-en/meditation/meditation-for-you/benefits-of-meditation

Kushi, Michio, and Alex Jack. *The Book of Macrobiotics*. Garden City Park, NY: Square One Publishers, 2012.

Kushi, Michio, and Alex Jack. *The Macrobiotic Path to Total Health*. New York: Ballantine Books, 2004.

Ober, Clinton, Stephen T. Sinatra, and Martin Zucker. *Earthing: The Most Important Health Discovery Ever*. Laguna Beach, CA: Basic Health Publications, 2014.

"Parasites That Can Lead to Cancer." American Cancer Society. Sep. 29, 2018. www.cancer.org/cancer/cancer-causes/infectious-agents/infections-that-can-lead-to-cancer/parasites.html

Stevenson, Shawn. "The Benefits of Earthing and Grounding: How Touching the Earth Can Improve Your Health." Conscious Lifestyle Magazine. Sep. 19, 2018. www.consciouslifestylemag.com/earthing-and-grounding-benefits

"Waking Up at the Same Time Each Night? The Chinese Medicine 'Body Clock' Explains Why." Turning Pointe Acupuncture and Wellness. February 19, 2017. www.turningpointeacu.com/blog/2017/2/19/waking-up-at-the-same-time-each-night-the-chinese-medicine-body-clock-explains-why

"Yeast Study Links Sugar to Growth of Cancer Cells." Community Research and Development Information Service. Dec. 21, 2017. https://cordis.europa.eu/news/rcn/128723/en

Zucker, Martin. "Earthing: Real Healing Power Right Under Your Feet." Manataka American Indian Council. Sep. 19, 2018. www.manataka.org/page2719.html

Chapter 11

"Cancer and the Environment." U.S. Department of Health and Human Services, National Institutes of Health, National Cancer Institute, National Institute of Environmental Health Sciences. Dec. 23, 2018. www.niehs.nih.gov/health/materials/cancer_and_the_environment_508.pdf

"Cancer Stat Facts: Statistics at a Glance." National Cancer Institute. Nov. 14, 2018. https://seer.cancer.gov/statfacts/html/all.html

"Farid Fata." Wikipedia. Oct. 4, 2018. https://en.wikipedia.org/wiki/Farid_Fata

"Harms of Cigarette Smoking and Health Benefits of Quitting." National Cancer Institute. Dec. 10, 2018. www.cancer.gov/about-cancer/causes-prevention/risk/tobacco/cessation-fact-sheet

"How Much Arsenic Is in Your Rice?" Consumer Reports. Nov. 18, 2014. www.consumerreports.org/cro/magazine/2015/01/how-much-arsenic-is-in-your-rice/index.htm

"Mold: The Common Toxin That Can Be FAR More Damaging Than Pesticides and Heavy Metals." Mercola. Sep. 3, 2011. https://articles.mercola.com/sites/articles/archive/2011/09/03/molds-making-you-ill.aspx

"Nagalase Test, Cancer Biomarker." Clinica biomedic. Jan. 1, 2019. www.biomedicenter.com/nagalase-test-cancer-biomarker

"Paint Exposure May Increase Cancer Risk." EHS Today. Mar. 19, 2002. www.ehstoday.com/news/ehs_imp_35288

Bollinger, Ty. "What Most Doctors REALLY Think About Alternative Cancer Treatments." The Truth About Cancer. Oct. 31, 2018. https://thetruthaboutcancer.com/doctors-really-think -alternative-cancer-treatments

Cowden, W. Lee, and Connie Strasheim. *Foods That Fit a Unique You*. Mill Valley, CA: ACIM Press, 2014.

Desaulniers, Veronique. "How Emotional Trauma Can Create Cancer . . . and 4 Ways to Stop It." The Truth About Cancer. Apr. 26, 2018. https://thetruthaboutcancer.com/emotional-trauma-cancer

Forster, Victoria. "A New $500 Blood Test Could Detect Cancer Before Symptoms Develop." Forbes. Jan. 18, 2018. www.forbes.com/sites/victoriaforster/2018/01/18/a-new-500-blood-te st-could-detect-cancer-before-symptoms-develop/#3d20cce17dd4

Frazier, Vidya. "Cordless Phone Radiation Danger," Earthcalm. June 1, 2011. https://shop.earthcalm.com/Cordless-Phone-Radiation-Danger_b_20.html

Gittleman, Ann Louise. "Join the Green Team," Ann Louise. Apr. 28, 2013. https://annlouise.com/2013/04/18/join-the-green-team

Gittleman, Ann Louise. *How to Stay Young and Healthy in a Toxic World*. New Canaan, CT: Keats Publishing, 1999.

Greer, Beth. *Super Natural Home*. Emmaus, PA: Rodale, 2009.

Joshi, Sumedha M. "The Sick Building Syndrome." *Indian J Occup Environ Med* 12, 2 (Aug. 2008): 61–64. doi: 10.4103/0019-5278.43262

Kamerud, Kristin L., Hobbie, Kevin A., and Kim A. Anderson. "Stainless Steel Leaches Nickel and Chromium into Foods During Cooking." *J. Agric. Food Chem*. 61, 39 (2013). 9495–9501. doi: 10.1021/jf402400v

Payer, Allyson. "The #1 Fabric to Avoid, According to Science." Who What Wear. Apr. 23, 2018. www.whowhatwear.com/worst-fabrics-for-skin

Singla, Veena. "Toxic Dust: The Dangerous Chemical Brew in Every Home," NRDC. Sep. 13, 2016. www.nrdc.org/experts/veena-singla/toxic-dust-dangerous-chemical-brew-every-home

Sipherd, Ray. "The Third-Leading Cause of Death in U.S. Most Doctors Don't Want You to Know About." CNBC. Feb. 22, 2018. www.cnbc.com/2018/02/22/medical-errors-third-leading-cause-of-death-in-america.html

Chapter 12

Duehring, Cindy. "Carpet Concerns: Carpet Installers Speak Out as the Medical Evidence Mounts," Inspired Living. Oct. 14, 2018. https://inspiredliving.com/airpurification/a~toxic-carpets2.htm

Erickson, Britt E. "How many chemicals are in use today?" c&en Global Enterprise. Feb. 27, 2017. https://pubs.acs.org/doi/abs/10.1021/cen-09509-govpol

Kippola, Palmer. "Top 6 Autoimmune Triggers: Infections." Beat Autoimmune. Oct. 16, 2018. www.beatautoimmune.com/infections/top-6-autoimmune-triggers-infections